Cooking with
Healing
Mushrooms

150 Delicious Adaptogen-Rich Recipes that Boost Immunity, Reduce Inflammation & Promote Whole Body Health

STEPFANIE ROMINE

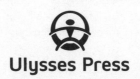

Ulysses Press

Text copyright © 2018 Stepfanie Romine. Design and concept copyright © 2018 Ulysses Press and its licensors. All rights reserved. Any unauthorized duplication in whole or in part or dissemination of this edition by any means (including but not limited to photocopying, electronic devices, digital versions, and the internet) will be prosecuted to the fullest extent of the law.

Published in the United States by:
ULYSSES PRESS
P.O. Box 3440
Berkeley, CA 94703
www.ulyssespress.com

ISBN: 978-1-61243-838-2
Library of Congress Control Number: 2018944069

Printed in Canada by Marquis Book Printing
10 9 8 7 6 5 4 3 2 1

Acquisitions editor: Bridget Thoreson
Managing editor: Claire Chun
Editor: Lauren Harrison
Proofreader: Shayna Keyles
Front cover design: Raquel Castro
Cover photos: front and spine © Victoria43/shutterstock.com; back © Africa
  Studio/shutterstock.com
Interior design: Jake Flaherty

Distributed by Publishers Group West

NOTE TO READERS: This book has been written and published strictly for informational and educational purposes only. It is not intended to serve as medical advice or to be any form of medical treatment. You should always consult your physician before altering or changing any aspect of your medical treatment and/or undertaking a diet regimen, including the guidelines as described in this book. Do not stop or change any prescription medications without the guidance and advice of your physician. Any use of the information in this book is made on the reader's good judgment after consulting with his or her physician and is the reader's sole responsibility. This book is not intended to diagnose or treat any medical condition and is not a substitute for a physician.

This book is independently authored and published and no sponsorship or endorsement of this book by, and no affiliation with, any trademarked brands or other products mentioned within is claimed or suggested. All trademarks that appear in ingredient lists and elsewhere in this book belong to their respective owners and are used here for informational purposes only. The author and publisher encourage readers to patronize the quality brands mentioned in this book.

To my mom, an extraordinary woman.

Contents

CHAPTER 6

Main Dishes 99

CHAPTER 7

Snacks 136

CHAPTER 8

Desserts 169

CHAPTER 9

Condiments, Flavorings, and Other Infusions 196

CHAPTER 10

Broths 207

CHAPTER 11

Drinks and Elixirs 217

A portion of the proceeds from this book will go to Bounty and Soul, a grassroots, volunteer-run nonprofit that provides healthy food, nutrition education, and other resources to underserved communities in Buncombe County, North Carolina, ensuring that health and healthy eating are not a luxury, but a right. All donations will go toward providing plant-based and, of course, mushroom-based foods! I am honored to help support the mission and values of Bounty and Soul.

Introduction

Growing up in a small Ohio town, I was exposed to mushrooms in exactly two contexts: canned on pizza or raw from salad bars. Neither one appealed to me, so I filed mushrooms away under "foods I don't like" until I became a vegetarian in the late '90s. Back then, if you didn't eat meat, your best option at a restaurant was usually a portobello mushroom sandwich. And so I learned to like mushrooms, one soggy, underseasoned, oversalted portobello at a time.

A few years later, I spent three months living in the Loire Valley in France. During my homestay and trips into Paris, I was introduced to other types of mushrooms: porcini, morels, and oysters, especially. Still, I never attempted to cook them myself. They seemed so exotic and gourmet—after all, that's how such mushrooms were labeled in U.S. supermarkets.

Then in 2005, I moved to South Korea to teach English. That vegetarian diet was a distant memory, and I had grown into an adventurous foodie. For 14 months, the South Korean capital of Seoul became my playground. Armed with my pocket dictionary and an eagerness to try new foods, I explored restaurants and markets every chance I had. Even a trip to the Carrefour supermarket around the corner from my high-rise apartment building was an adventure. Mushrooms were an integral part of the Korean diet, from shiitake and enoki to plain buttons and velvety oysters.

At the end of every term, my coworkers and I gathered for a celebratory dinner. It was often Korean barbecue, with rich meats cooked over charcoal in a humble streetside stall. But in the bitter cold winter months, we chose *shabu shabu*, pots of boiling mushroom and beef broth served with thin slices of raw beef, ruffly Napa cabbage leaves, and an assortment of mushrooms.

The dish was simple and communal—like so many of my most memorable meals in Seoul—and those mushrooms were what captured my attention. Jars of them lined the counter at the restaurant, and the servers would trim off the fruiting bodies moments before serving them. We'd plunge the mushrooms into the boiling broth, then eat them with a variety of spicy and savory sauces. I'd never seen enoki mushrooms before, and they seemed otherworldly, little pearls atop delicate strands. I had no idea then that mushrooms were medicinal.

The transition from mushrooms as a culinary delight to medicinal ingredient happened years later, after I moved to the mountains of North Carolina in search of a simpler life. I'm not sure I ever would have written this cookbook if I hadn't moved to Asheville back in 2012. Before then, I cooked with mushrooms only for flavor, and my "favorite" mushroom was likely a truffle. But here in the Blue Ridge Mountains, mushrooms have a way of finding you and drawing you in to their magic, their medicine, and their beauty. A few months after moving here, my now husband, Sam, and I found ourselves at the Asheville City Market. Going to the farmers' market (and sometimes more than one) had long been a weekend ritual for me, but this one was so different from the ones I knew up north. The Asheville market had the usual locally sourced vegetables, meats, and baked goods, but it also had nearly a dozen vendors selling herbal elixirs, tinctures, and dried ingredients I didn't recognize.

One of those vendors was Alan Muskat, a mycologist and forager who through his company No Place Like Home leads wild edible hunting trips year-round in the forests and valleys surrounding Asheville. Alan's table was a dizzying display of new-to-me ingredients, which I sampled and savored with great enthusiasm. It was early yet, the market slow, and Alan had ample time to talk, which I would soon learn was a rarity, as his booth is quite popular.

Though I immediately forgot the names of each leaf he handed me, I felt emboldened with every bitter, astringent bite. We had moved to the mountains to live a healthier life more in touch with nature, and this, I smugly believed, was bringing me closer. "Look at me," I thought. "I'm eating wild native plants. I'm such an adventurous, eco-minded foodie!" (I tend to get carried away and go all in when something strikes my fancy.) Then I tried a fragrant spruce tip, its piney taste overwhelming my taste buds. I felt like I was trying to eat a car air freshener. I tried not to cough as I struggled to swallow it. I took a huge swig of water and prepared to make my exit, realizing it was only six weeks ago that I had been living in a walk-up apartment in the gritty urban core of Cincinnati, not a tiny house with a wood stove nestled against a mountainside in the dense treetop canopy. I had a long way to go before I would be ready to trust myself in nature.

Then I saw it: a lacquered, mahogany-striped object sitting in the middle of the table. I hadn't a clue what it was, but I was in awe of its beauty. I ran my fingers over its smooth, striated surface and admired the natural ombre pattern, from deep rust to eggshell. Surely, this came from nature, but what was it? I inquired with Alan. He explained that it was reishi, a type of medicinal mushroom readily found in the nearby forests. I was in love. I wanted to learn more, not only about this mysterious mushroom that looked and felt more like insulation than any mushrooms I knew, but also about the plants and animals with whom I shared a habitat.

After that encounter, I joined an herbal community-shared agriculture program, called Herban Farmacy, paying a monthly fee in exchange for several handcrafted herbal medicines. Each month, I eagerly awaited my trip into town to pick up my goodies and chat with Jamie, the owner, who also happened to hail from Ohio. The ingredients list on every tea blend, tincture, and salve read like a foreign language to me, and I eagerly researched each plant and mushroom, asking Jamie about them and reading anything I could get my hands on.

Stinging nettles, I learned, were traditionally used to treat seasonal allergies, and I recalled having bought some several years prior. Black elderberry, which I had tried in jams and beverages during trips to Europe, was for immune system health. And one month there was a tincture with reishi, that beautiful mushroom that had enchanted me at Alan's booth.

This mushroom, I discovered, was found across several continents and had been used for its healing properties for thousands of years. In traditional Chinese medicine (TCM), it was even known as "the mushroom of immortality." Though it would be another few years before I heard the term "adaptogen," a friend explained that reishi could help with stress—a constant battle in my life—as well as sleep. I took that tincture to the last drop!

Herbs and mushrooms became my hobby, one that paired well with running, which had become much more of a struggle due to hilly terrain and higher elevation. To pass the time as I slowly logged the miles to train for my first mountainous half-marathon, I gazed at the flora and, less often, the fauna, surrounding me. I noticed elder bushes, with their lacy flowers that would ripen into immune-boosting berries. I spied ruby-red clusters of sumac, which I knew could be made into a tasty lemonade-like drink. And sometimes I spotted mushrooms. I was always on the lookout for reishi, but they eluded me. (I later learned I needed to look up, not down, to see them!)

A longtime plant-based eater, I started to awaken to the idea that plants could not only nourish and fuel me; they could heal me as well. (I didn't yet differentiate between plants and mushrooms, since in the culinary sense, they're lumped in with vegetables.) And so, the seed was sown—I was hooked by the world of natural healing. I became so enamored of herbalism that I started to research certification programs. They were beyond my budget just then—and the best ones had waiting lists for at least a year—so I kept up my self-study. Then, fate struck: I ended up working for a large herbal supplements manufacturer. I would be their copywriter and get paid to learn about herbs, then write about them!

For the next three years, I dove head-first into soaking up all I could from the experts who surrounded me. I attended trade shows and herbal conferences, rubbed elbows with pioneers in the resurgence of herbal medicine, and had the great fortune of working closely with naturopath, renowned herbalist, and author Dr. Mary Bove, one of the most knowledgeable and also kindest and most generous humans I've ever met. I also got paid to learn to cook with herbs.

During my first year on the job, I cohosted dinners at the company farmhouse kitchen, first with the founder and later with the corporate chef. We cooked with herbs, of course, and often mushrooms—sometimes shiitakes that I got to help harvest. As part of that project, I researched ayurveda and traditional Chinese medicine, and devoured every pearl of wisdom I could. It was there I first tried wood ear mushrooms—I found them somewhat bland but developed an affinity for them because they reminded me of the capsules that miraculously bloomed into brightly colored, fun-shaped sponges that I had played with as a kid. You'll see what I mean the first time you reconstitute dried wood ears.

My last project with Mary and my team was researching the very healing mushrooms that are the subject of this book. From turkey tail to reishi, lion's mane to chaga, I immersed myself in the world of fungi. For the better part of a year, I pored over research and every book I could find on mushrooms as medicine. I began cooking with them more frequently—and not just the everyday varieties like buttons and portobellos. I got to spend hours on conference calls with world-renowned mycologists, learning how to find the best-quality mushrooms and how best to prepare them.

My time with the company drew to an end, as I transitioned to writing full time, but my passion for mushrooms and herbs has only strengthened. In 2016, my husband and I moved into a tiny cottage on the edge of a historic 23-acre property. The driveway, the oldest existing stone road in North Carolina, is lined with towering hemlocks, so each summer I can see from my front door burnt-orange reishi fruiting bodies stuck out from tree trunks like natural awnings. Deep in the woods, I discovered a cache of morels our first spring, and in summer, vibrant orange cinnabar chanterelles greet me along my runs. (I've learned to run with a spare bag throughout summer and fall, for spontaneous mushroom hunts.)

And, as I sit here writing, I can see a patch of turkey tails that overtook an old stump. I've grown oyster mushrooms in my kitchen, and driven an hour out of my way to procure a box of organic lion's mane mushrooms. I've tinctured my own immune mushroom blends and made every treat and meal imaginable with them.

So when the opportunity to write an entire book on healing mushrooms presented itself to me, it was a dream come true. As someone who wasn't raised with much exposure to holistic or natural health, discovering the power of nature has been transformative. I firmly believe in the healing benefits of mushrooms as a functional superfood. I hope this book conveys how easy, affordable, and rewarding it can be to integrate mushrooms into your health and wellness routines.

I'm a cookbook author, certified health coach, and fitness nutrition specialist with continuing education in ayurveda, herbal supplements, and holistic and integrative nutrition. I am also a trained journalist. For this book, I interviewed mycologists and naturopathic doctors, dietitians and mushroom "farmers." I teamed up with friend and fellow Western North Carolina writer Abby Artemisia, a well-respected botanist, herbalist, and forager, for some of the more traditional recipes. I also sought input from these experts on some of my own creations.

While I am passionate and knowledgeable about medicinal mushrooms and natural health, I want to be clear that I am not prescribing or diagnosing for any condition or ailment. Please consult your health care professional before starting any new supplement.

The recipes in this book are designed to help you integrate mushrooms into your daily diet, not to treat, diagnose, treat, cure, or prevent any disease or health condition.

Think of it like this: Eating mushrooms as part of a healthy, whole foods diet is like squirreling away $20 from each paycheck you earn. It doesn't take much effort, but it builds up over time. However, if you're in debt or close to retirement, those $20 contributions won't make much of a dent in your debt or be enough to live on in your later years. If you're interested in taking mushrooms therapeutically, such as in the doses used in clinical studies, talk to a naturopath or registered dietitian. You *can* have too much of a good thing. If you ate enough shiitakes, for example, to reach the clinical therapeutic dose of lentinan, you'd end up with a major bellyache—and some unsavory GI side effects.

Nature takes her time, and so do mushrooms. While you need to consult with your health care professional for the correct dosage for you, a general rule is to allow at least one season (three months or so) and up to nine months for a mushroom or herb to take its full effect.

CHAPTER 1

Why Mushrooms?

The entire time I was writing this cookbook, people asked: "Why mushrooms?" "Why not?" was my immediate response, before I explained my passion for cooking with fungi. There are 38,000 species of fungi globally, and we know of 2,000 that are edible.[1] However, most of us have tried just a few: portobello/cremini/white and perhaps shiitake or porcini. But there's a whole world of mushrooms out there (quite literally), so if you've written off mushrooms like I did as a kid, I implore you to give them another try. (And, since you're reading this, you likely either have or are considering it.)

In 2000, Americans consumed 2.5 pounds of portobello/cremini/white mushrooms annually per capita. By 2017, we were eating 20 percent more of those 'shrooms.[2] And that doesn't count all the wild and exotic mushrooms that are more readily available than they were even a decade ago. We're getting into mushrooms in the kitchen—and we're using them as medicine more often too, says Dr. Bove. "Mushrooms have gotten more popular and more understood," she said. We've even learned that mushrooms are actually closer to humans than plants are, if you compare DNA.[3]

When Dr. Bove began practicing herbalism more than 40 years ago, medicinal herbs were not found on grocery store shelves, and few species of mushrooms were readily available either. As we've collectively started to return to our roots and rediscover the value of holistic and natural healing practices, we've also embraced medicinal and healing herbs—a definition that includes the greater plant kingdom as well as mushrooms and other fungi such as lichen.

"Many people don't think about mushrooms as herbs—they think of them as food," says Bove. "But they do act like a medicinal plant, like a medicinal herb. I like that people call them *medicinal* mushrooms now."

This mushroom renaissance comes at an important time for us as a society, says Bove. In addition to the influx of good-quality extracts on the market, she says, mushrooms are "effective and poignant for our current time and needs." Our neuroendocrine systems are breaking down—we're sick and we're stressed and we're sick of being stressed.

The 2017 Stress in America survey from the American Psychological Association found that nearly two-thirds of Americans believe this is the lowest point in history that they can remember.[4] In addition, 66 percent are worried about their health and the cost of health insurance.[5] The real kicker? Stress interferes with immune function, so we're creating a vicious cycle.[6]

Anxiety disorders are the most common mental illness in the U.S., affecting 40 million adults annually, and we're in the middle of an autoimmune epidemic.[7, 8] And though a 2016 review in the journal *BMC Endocrine Disorders* called adrenal fatigue a myth, anyone who's dealt with chronic stress knows how hard it can be to recover from stress-related fatigue and overwhelm.[9] As a yoga teacher, I regularly witness how reconnecting with the breath and breaking the cycle of stress impacts every other aspect of someone's life—including the immune system.

I dealt with chronic stress myself last year. I found myself on edge, forgetful, and exhausted. In the span of six months, I had a lingering respiratory infection, influenza A, bronchitis, and several colds (all of which I treated with herbal and other holistic methods under the guidance of a naturopath). It took months to regain my usual energy and immune health, during which time I leaned heavily on adaptogens, including mushrooms.

Mushrooms aren't magic—I preface most of my talks with that statement—but I believe they are time-honored and effective medicine.

Treat them with respect and reverence, and they'll do right by you. (And always take them under the supervision of a trained medical professional.)

The Anatomy and Life Cycle of Mushrooms

Mushrooms appear as if by magic, sprouting up from the forest floor or from the bark of trees seemingly overnight. Watch a time-lapse video of mushrooms growing, and you'll see why they're part of fairy and magic folklore. Their growth rates seem supernatural, or like something out of an animated film.

Most of the magic happens behind the scenes; what we know as a mushroom is often just a small part of the organism and one step in the life cycle. These fruiting bodies (what we tend to call "mushrooms") are near the end of a mushroom's life cycle, and they are visible for just a few days—then they disappear into the ether just as before.

Mushrooms start as spores, which are akin to seeds for plants. In nature, spores are carried on the wind or another organism until they find a favorable place to grow. Each species of mushrooms requires a certain host or substrate. Just as you can't grow a palm tree in Alaska, mushrooms need specific climates, soil, trees, etc.

These spores start to grow into mycelium, which are like the roots of a mushroom. The mycelium collects and utilizes nutrients from the soil and surrounding environment, and also fights off predators by releasing enzymes and other protective constituents. Mycelium is kind of like the mushroom's immune system.

The mycelium eventually grows into tiny mushrooms, which mature into the fruiting body or bodies. The fruiting bodies produce and release spores, and the life cycle starts all over again.

Mushroom Lexicon

Cap: The top of a mushroom fruiting body.

Fruiting body: This is what we think of when we think "mushrooms"—it's the above-ground part of a mushroom you can see. This is the part that produces the spores.

Fungi: The kingdom to which mushrooms belong. Includes molds, rusts, mildews, smuts, mushrooms, and yeasts.

Gills: The ridges under the cap of some mushroom fruiting bodies, used to disperse spores.

Mushroom: Fruiting body, or the part of the mushroom that grows above the ground or outside of a tree.

Mycelium (singular) or mycelia (plural): The "roots" of a mushroom. They collect and utilize nutrients.

Mycology: The study of fungi.

Mycologist: One who studies fungi.

Spores: The "seeds" or reproductive parts of a mushroom. These float through the air, seemingly invisible, then take root and turn into a mushroom.

Stalk: The stem of a mushroom fruiting body.

Traditionally, we have consumed the fruiting bodies of mushrooms. After all, the fruiting body is what most of us consider to be a mushroom. The mycelium (aka the roots) also has some medicinal value; you'll find mycelium in many mushroom supplements and powders.

Of the mushrooms in this cookbook, there is one exception: Chaga is actually a sclerotia, which is a hardened mycelial mass. The "mushroom" is hardly ever seen in nature, and what we know to be chaga is this dark brown or black mass.

Historic Uses of Mushrooms

The use of mushrooms as medicine started in the East, says Becky Beyer, an ethnobotanist and forager who is completing her master's degree in Appalachian studies at Appalachian State University in Boone, North Carolina. She teaches Appalachian folk medicine, and she says there's no mention of mushrooms as medicine in that lineage, though she knows the Cherokee did use mushrooms.

"A lot of what we are learning is a revival of other practices," like traditional Chinese medicine, says Beyer. Mushrooms have been used in China and across Asia for 7,000 years, and they are part of the classic early TCM text *The Yellow Emperor's Classic of Medicine*. Ancient TCM revered both reishi and cordyceps—they are considered tonics, the "highest class of medicines," as they promote longevity and strength. Not uncoincidentally, these two mushrooms are still among the most commonly used in TCM.[10] (In the West, Hippocrates used them to treat the kidneys around 455 BC.[11])

Our connection to mushrooms runs even deeper: Dating back as far as 6000 BC, the Tassili n'Ajjer cave paintings discovered in Algeria may depict humans holding mushrooms, wrote Terrance McKenna in his 1993 book *Food of the Gods: The Search for the Original Tree of Knowledge, A Radical History of Plants, Drugs, and Human Evolution*. And the prehistoric "iceman" discovered in the Alps in 1991 carried bracket fungi for medicine![12]

Modern Mushroom Medicine

We still prefer to eat our mushrooms—according to the Mushroom Council, we mostly consume white button, followed by cremini, portobellos, enoki, oyster, maitake, and shiitake.[13] But mushrooms as medicine are catching on, both as functional foods and as adaptogens (more on those later).[14]

Throughout her decades of practice, Bove has expanded her use of mushrooms. She has long used shiitake, reishi, maitake, and cordyceps, and a decade ago, she started to include turkey tail, chaga, and lion's mane as well. (All of those mushrooms are in Chapter 2.)

Beyer's glad to see more people getting in tune with the medicine nature has provided us. "Mushrooms to us are gifts," she said. "They're this other being that holds these insanely intricate compounds that have strange stories and folklore. They provide this comfort and mystery that humans find really attractive."

Walk into any Whole Foods, and you'll see how our interest has mushroomed. The produce section boasts varieties from enoki to shiitake, while the supplements section has powders, capsules, and tinctures galore. There's mushroom coffee, mushroom chocolate, and mushroom jerky. We've come a long way from those soggy jarred mushrooms!

Mushroom Nutrition

Since we mostly eat mushrooms—and this is a healing mushrooms cookbook, after all—let's first look the nutrition of mushrooms. Mushrooms have tremendous nutritional value. Though they're mostly water, they provide plenty of nutrients: protein, B vitamins, complex carbohydrates, fiber, minerals like selenium and copper, and various antioxidants, including ergothioneine and glutathione. Due to their high water content, mushrooms are nutrient-dense but not calorically dense, so they are frequently touted for their ability to help you stay fuller for fewer calories and less fat.[19] Mushrooms contain almost no fat and are low in sodium. Since they are not animal products, they do not contain cholesterol, and they're naturally vegan and gluten-free.

Nutritional Highlights of Mushrooms

Protein: Mushrooms are high in protein and provide most essential amino acids.[20] Mushrooms in general provide 1 to 2 grams of protein per cup.[21] While that seems skimpy compared with meat, mushrooms are high in protein by percentage of their weight, and that protein is quite digestible too.[22] Individual species vary, but not enough that it's worth prioritizing one over another for that reason.

Vitamin D: Mushrooms are the only non-animal food source that contains vitamin D. They "make" the sunshine vitamin much in the same way we do: Mushrooms absorb sunlight, then convert it to vitamin D. They contain a plant sterol called ergosterol that, when exposed to UV light, converts to vitamin D2.[23]

Some growers expose their mushrooms to UV light, which increases their vitamin D content. For example, when exposed to UV light, a grilled portobello contains as much vitamin D as a 3-ounce portion of sockeye salmon![24]

B vitamins: Another rarity among non-animal foods, mushrooms also contain several B vitamins, including riboflavin, niacin, and B12.[25]

Antioxidants: Antioxidants protect the body from free radical damage and reduce systemic inflammation and chronic disease (think of them like the body's fire extinguishers or sprinkler systems).

The selenium in mushrooms may promote heart health and reduce cancer risks.[26] Selenium is an essential mineral and antioxidant that helps with thyroid function, antioxidant support, and DNA production.

Ergothioneine is a naturally occurring antioxidant found in mushrooms that may help protect the body's cells.[27] Certain species (porcini and some oysters) are higher than others in both ergothioneine and another potent antioxidant called glutathione, but mushrooms in general are considered to be the richest food source of ergothioneine.[28]

Mushrooms have also been shown in studies to:

- Positively impact blood sugar levels after meals.[29]

- Help mitigate the risk of developing type-2 diabetes in older, at-risk individuals.[30]

- Reduce the risk of breast cancer and dementia, according to observational studies (which do not prove causal relationships).[31]

- Offer "immunomodulatory, lipid-lowering, antitumor, and other beneficial or therapeutic health effects without any significant toxicity."[32]

In addition, mushrooms are known for providing essential vitamins and minerals. The chart below lists just a few mushrooms known for their nutrient contents. A food that is an "excellent" source of a nutrient contains 20 percent of the Daily Value. A "good" source contains 10 to 20 percent of the Daily Value.

	NUTRITION HIGHLIGHTS[33]
Button mushroom	Good source: selenium, B vitamins (riboflavin, niacin and pantothenic acid), and copper.
Cremini	Excellent source: selenium, riboflavin, and copper. Good source: phosphorus, niacin, and pantothenic acid.
Enoki	Excellent source: niacin. Good source: riboflavin and pantothenic acid.
Maitake	Good source: copper, riboflavin, and niacin.
Oyster mushroom	Excellent source: niacin. Good source: copper, riboflavin, and pantothenic acid.
Portobello	Excellent source: selenium. Good source: phosphorus, copper, and niacin.
Shiitake	Excellent source: copper, selenium, and pantothenic acid. Good source: niacin.

Cook Your Mushrooms

I love seeing mushrooms on menus and in my Instagram feed, but there's one common mistake I see from chefs and home cooks alike: raw mushrooms! Please, please, please stop eating raw mushrooms—especially the white buttons. First of all, they're spongy and weird. But more importantly, you're wasting your money and not getting the most nutrition from your 'shrooms.

The cell walls of mushrooms are made mostly of a material called chitin, which is indigestible. This is the same material that makes up fish scales, insect exoskeletons, and crustacean shells. The good news is that cooking breaks down chitin (and protein), and it increases starch, total dietary fiber, and fat, so more of those nutrients are made available to our bodies.[15] Chitin content is higher in older mushrooms, so a portobello contains more than a cremini, for example.

In addition, wild and cultivated mushrooms contain a compound called agaritine, which has been identified as a potential carcinogen. While a 2010 review in the *Journal of Functional Foods* determined that our consumption of "cultivated *A. bisporus* mushrooms poses no known toxicological risk to healthy humans," the general consensus remains that cooked mushrooms are better.[16] Mushrooms do contain some antinutrients, so don't eat them raw! Raw mushrooms can interfere with protein absorption and may cause small lesions in the small intestine.[17]

Eating raw shiitakes specifically can cause a toxic reaction that leaves a rash like dermatitis in some individuals; the North American Mycological Association advises that you always cook shiitakes thoroughly.[18] Interestingly enough, it is the anti-cancer component lentinan that causes the rash!

Raw or undercooked morels are toxic, so always cook them thoroughly and in a well-ventilated area.

Mushrooms and Immune Health

Mushrooms contain numerous types of carbohydrates, including starch and a type of complex carbohydrate (polysaccharide) called beta-glucans. These beta-glucans have been shown to stimulate the immune system and inhibit tumor growth. Certain mushrooms have specific polysaccharides, such as the lentinan found in shiitakes or PSK in turkey tails. Mushrooms also contain components including terpenes and steroids that have anti-tumor activity.[34] Other active components include hericenones in lion's mane and cordycepin in cordyceps.

Beta-glucans are also found in the cell walls of lichens, grains, and sea vegetables. They are named based on their branching structure; mushrooms have beta-glucans 1 through 6. Beta-glucans naturally increase and stimulate antibodies and natural killer cells (they limit the spread and damage of certain types of infections and tumors), and they influence gene expression and healthy cell growth (in other words, they have anti-cancer properties). This is why all the mushrooms in this book are considering to be immunosupportive.

In the spring 2017 issue of *HerbalGram: The Journal of the American Botanical Council*, renowned herbalist and mycologist Christopher Hobbs explained how beta-glucans work in the body. (Hobbs cited 122 studies on the safety and efficacy of medicinal mushrooms— the research out there is astounding!)

After ingesting mushrooms, beta-glucans bind with macrophages (a type of white blood cell that consumes and breaks down cellular debris) in the intestines. From there, the beta-glucans are ingested and transported to the spleen, lymph nodes, and bone marrow, among other sites. In the marrow, the beta-glucans are further broken down, giving them "an enhanced ability to kill tumor cells."[35]

Some mushrooms—which you'll learn about in the next chapter—are immune stimulants, directly working on the immune system to boost defenses against specific stresses like viruses and bacteria.[36] These immune stimulants increase activity of macrophages. Cordyceps, shiitake, and turkey tail provide this type of support.

Other mushrooms are immune tonics, meaning they support, nourish, and strengthen the system in general, or specific parts like bone marrow (the source of all macrophages and other immune cells) or red blood cells. Immune-tonifying mushrooms include reishi, cordyceps, and shiitake.

Mushrooms as Adaptogens

Adaptogens are plants (and mushrooms) that observe the Hippocratic Oath: First do no harm. These herbs, as first defined by Soviet physician and scientist Nikolai Lazarev in 1947, add no stress to the body, help the body adapt to both environmental and psychological stresses, and have a nonspecific response in the body (resistance to stressors), supporting all major systems including the nervous, endocrine, and immune systems.[37] They can also regulate bodily functions like blood sugar. By 1985, researchers had discovered that adaptogens also support adrenal function (meaning they help the body cope with stress, which is likely why you've heard of them).

Adaptogens directly support the immune system to build the body's defenses to nonspecific stresses—chemicals/toxins, noise, overwork, etc. Within the immune system, adaptogens support and balance the endocrine system so that it does not impair our natural defenses.

Herbs like tulsi (holy basil), ginseng, eleuthero, and licorice are adaptogens, as are cordyceps and reishi mushrooms. (To learn more about adaptogens, read David Winston's book of the same name.)[38] Adaptogens are super trendy right now, but they've been used for centuries in Russia and China.

Beyond offering stress and immune support, here are some other areas of the body where mushrooms might offer benefits.

Beauty

- Chaga
- Cordyceps
- Enoki
- King Trumpet
- Lion's Mane
- Maitake
- Shiitake
- Turkey Tail

Blood Sugar/Healthy Weight

- Chaga
- Maitake
- Oyster
- Reishi

Detox/Liver

- Cordyceps
- Enoki
- King Trumpet
- Oyster
- Reishi
- Shiitake
- Turkey Tail

Digestive/GI Health

- Lion's mane
- Maitake
- Wood ear

Endurance/Performance/Recovery

- Cordyceps
- King Trumpet
- Maitake
- Reishi

Energy

- Cordyceps
- King Trumpet
- Lion's Mane
- Maitake
- Reishi
- Turkey Tail

Heart Health/Cholesterol

- King Trumpet
- Maitake
- Oyster
- Reishi
- Shiitake

Memory/Cognition

- Cordyceps
- Lion's Mane
- Reishi

Stress

- Chaga
- Cordyceps
- Maitake
- Oyster
- Reishi

CHAPTER 2

Major and Minor Mushrooms for Medicine

Choosing a favorite mushroom would be tough for me to do; I value each one that I've included in this book for its unique flavor, nutrition, and potential health benefits. That said, some mushrooms have been studied more than others, and some have shown more significant results than the rest.

For this cookbook, I've categorized the mushrooms as major and minor to distinguish those that have been extensively studied and are well-documented as adaptogens and immune modulators or stimulators. NPR called mushrooms "the superheroes of the fungi kingdom," and as with, say, the Marvel or DC Comics rosters, there are some individuals that simply get more attention.[39] If you're just trying to eat more mushrooms as part of an overall healthy diet, this distinction isn't very important. Just eat more mushrooms! But, if you're looking for specific mushrooms to support a certain aspect of your health, perhaps as directed by your acupuncturist or naturopath, you might be more interested in the specific health benefits of each species.

The major mushrooms are chaga, cordyceps, enoki, lion's mane, maitake, oyster, reishi, shiitake, and turkey tail. The minor mushrooms are either less studied or simply have been shown to offer general immune support. They include boletes (also known as cèpe or porcini mushrooms), chanterelle, king trumpet, morel, white button (including the related cremini and portobello), and wood ear, along with any other edible mushroom.

For each mushroom, I've shared a general overview along with both traditional and evidence-based uses. Traditional use—like the thousands of years of use in Eastern herbalism practices like TCM—may be sufficient for you. For those who prefer studies and research, I've cited studies when appropriate, and I encourage you to read Robert Rogers's *The Fungal Pharmacy: The Complete Guide to Medicinal Mushrooms and Lichens of North America* or Christopher Hobbs' *Medicinal Mushrooms: An Exploration of Tradition, Healing, and Culture* (both of which are my primary reference books for all things fungi). Both of these authors are expert herbalists and mycologists who bring mushroom medicine to life. And then there is Paul Stamets—read any of his books (*Mycelium Running* is my top pick and was the first mushroom book I ever read) or watch his TED Talk to get excited about mushrooms.

Let's get to know these healing mushrooms. The primers in this chapter will introduce you to each of the mushrooms used in my recipes. I should note that just because a mushroom isn't in this cookbook doesn't mean it lacks medicinal qualities. There are 2,000 edible mushrooms that we know of, after all!

Major Medicinal Mushrooms

The major mushrooms have longer descriptions than the minor mushrooms because they tend to be used more for their healing potential and adaptogenic qualities than for their flavor, with a few exceptions (shiitake, maitake, and oysters). Several of these mushrooms are tough and grow on trees, so they must be consumed as extracts. We'll delve into the tough and tender mushrooms in Chapter 3.

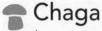 Chaga

Inonotus obliquus

Also known as: Cinder or birch conk, clinker polypore, black gold

Common uses: Antioxidant protection and immune health

Chaga looks like a chunk of burned wood—you'd never guess it's actually a mushroom. That's because the fruiting body of this tonic mushroom is rarely seen and not used medicinally. We use the sclerotia (also known as the canker), which is a hardened mycelial mass that intertwines with the host—essentially, chaga infects a birch tree and eventually kills it. The sclerotia is basically a tumor, which is fascinating considering chaga's traditional use in treating tumors! Commonly found in Eastern Europe and North America, chaga is traditionally considered to be a blood purifier and pain reliever with potent antioxidant properties. It has a long history of traditional use for cancer, particularly in Russian folk medicine.

Its active components (triterpenoids) depend on precursor substances drawn from its host, birch trees. Chaga inhibits NFKB, a protein that turns inflammation on and off in the body (think of it like a smoke detector for inflammation).

Cordyceps

Cordyceps sinensis, Cordyceps militaris

Also known as: Winter worm, vegetable caterpillar, Chinese caterpillar fungus

Common uses: Adaptogen; energy, stamina, and endurance; immune health

What a time to be alive! This mushroom was so highly valued in imperial China that we commoners wouldn't have been allowed to have cordyceps, even if we could afford it.

It was used to increase stamina and vital energy in ancient China, which is one reason why cordyceps has gained a reputation among athletes.[40] My husband, an avid cyclist, brought home a bottle of cordyceps capsules years before I had ever heard of this mushroom. A fellow racer swore by cordyceps supplements to give him an edge in tough criteriums—my husband won several races in his category that year, so that sold him on cordyceps.

Chances are, your cordyceps are vegan and did not take the lives of any innocent caterpillars. Since they must grow from a certain type of caterpillar, wild cordyceps sinensis are rare and pricey. Those wild mushrooms, *Cordyceps sinensis,* are rare and pricey. However, there is a more affordable, cultivated version that is vegan and more widely available. If you have the cash for it and can find the *sinensis,* go for it. However, the two species listed above are interchangeable and are both used in TCM.

As an adaptogen and a tonifying herb in TCM, cordyceps has a laundry list of traditional and modern uses. It is used in herbalism much like ginseng is, to boost stamina and restore energy, especially after you've been sick or exhausted. Cordyceps is also used to support healthy aging—and a healthy sex drive! Cordycepin is its best-known active component.

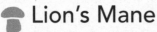 Lion's Mane

Hericium erinaceus

Also known as: Hedgehog mushroom
Common uses: Memory, concentration, and nerve health

According to the Doctrine of Signatures, an herbalism practice dating back to the ancient Greeks, herbs resemble the body parts God intended for them to treat. Any guesses what lion's mane would treat?

This shaggy mushroom is a nootropic, meaning it's a cognitive enhancer. Lion's mane helps creativity, motivation, and memory, as well as brain function. (Guess which mushroom I consumed regularly while working on deadline to write this book?)

Native to Europe, Asia, and North America (including where I live), lion's mane is unique in that it crosses the blood-brain barrier to directly support the brain and nervous system. It also stimulates nerve growth factor and has been used to treat various brain and nervous system ailments, including some degenerative conditions like dementia.[41] Because of its impact on the brain, this is another mushroom favored by athletes. In TCM, it is used for digestion, including gastric ulcers, and as a tonic for general malaise and lethargy.

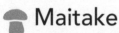 # Maitake
Grifola frondosa

Also known as: Hen of the woods, dancing mushrooms
Common uses: GI tract, blood sugar, and healthy weight

Maitake may be my favorite mushroom to eat (along with lion's mane). I do a little dance in my seat every time I taste the seared maitake from the Asheville restaurant Plant, so they really are a dancing mushroom to me! They earned the name dancing mushroom because maitake were so valued in feudal Japan that they were worth their weight in silver. So, when people discovered the mushrooms, they had hit pay dirt—of course they'd do a happy dance!

Commonly found in the eastern U.S., Europe, and Asia, these were only available in the wild until 1979, when they were successfully cultivated. As is common with cultivated mushrooms, the maitake you get at the grocery store have a milder taste and are more tender than those found in the wild.

In addition to immune support, these mushrooms have been shown to help lower blood glucose levels, and non-human studies have shown promise in using maitake for liver protection, blood pressure, and cholesterol.

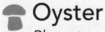 # Oyster

Pleurotus ostreatus

Also known as: Angel wings

Common uses: Cholesterol, immune health

"If anyone's going to call something a superfood, I think oyster mushrooms are it," said Nate Burrows, a mushroom enthusiast and sous chef at Plant restaurant in Asheville. I agree. These mushrooms, which grow on deciduous trees in North America, Europe, and Asia, are incredibly nutritious and delicious, and they come in vibrant shades of pink, yellow, white, brown, blue, and gray.

"Nutritionally speaking, the oyster mushroom falls between a high-grade vegetable and a low-grade meat when considered for biological value," wrote Rogers in *The Fungal Pharmacy*, and Hobbs raves about their protein and B-vitamin content in his book.

Oysters—whose name refers to their appearance, not their taste—have long been used as a nerve tonic and to lower cholesterol, particularly in Eastern Europe.[42] Lovastatin, a statin drug used to lower cholesterol, naturally occurs in oyster mushrooms. In TCM, oysters are used for joint and muscle relaxation and as a blood builder. They're an ingredient in "tendon-easing powder," which is used to treat low-back pain, among other ailments. Add oyster mushrooms to your dinner after a hard workout.

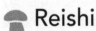 # Reishi

Ganoderma lucidum

Also known as: The mushroom of immortality; Queen of Mushrooms; ling zhi (spirit plant); here in western North Carolina, it is called white butt rock; *lucidum* means shiny/brilliant!

Common uses: Adaptogen; longevity, sleep, and immune health

If there's one mushroom to rule them all, it's reishi (pronounced RAY-shee; I called it REE-shee for years). Reishi protects the immune system by regulating natural killer cells and cytokine responses. Reishi is also a potent antioxidant that keeps inflammation in check.

"Reishi is the patron saint of our household," says Becky Beyer. She lives in an intentional community of seven outside of Asheville, and part of her contribution is teaching the others to forage for plants and mushrooms. "We forage so much reishi. There's always a pot of reishi tea on the stove. Whenever people come over, there's always some to give people."

Of all the mushrooms in this book, reishi is perhaps the most versatile, with 4,000 years of use in China and Japan. It can be bitter, which is a sign of its potency, as its triterpenes (one of the active components) naturally taste bitter. Beyond its common use for sleep, stress management, and general immune health and vitality, reishi has been used to support the liver and kidneys, as well as mediate high blood pressure, arthritis, bronchitis, asthma, gastric ulcers, cancer, and age-related decline. It's often used in TCM like ginseng is, to support endurance and balance endocrine and hormonal levels.[43] It's also used to soothe the skin and ease digestive issues. Dr. Bove calls reishi a restorative adaptogen, and it seems to have a relaxing effect throughout the body, relieving the tension that stress creates both physically and emotionally.

Mushrooms and Cancer

I want to make this explicitly clear: A stir-fry isn't going to cure cancer. Neither is a smoothie. When mushrooms are used in cancer treatments, patients are not told to eat them daily or put them in their coffee. They are given specific extracts that often isolate an active constituent.

Cancer treatments contain concentrated doses of substances like lentinan or LEM from shiitake, or the PSK from turkey tails. When we consume mushrooms, we're building our bank account and investing in a healthy future—it's not like hitting the lottery and paying off all your debts at once. In most cases, you would need to eat so many mushrooms to have the same therapeutic effect of extracts that it would definitely cause GI upset and potentially toxicity.

Reishi ranges in color from reddish orange to black, and it grows across the U.S., Europe, South America, and Asia. It grows well on elm, alder, oak, and some conifers. The price of reishi has declined in the last few decades, as it can now be cultivated.

Why These Aren't "Magic" Mushrooms

We are a society that desperately wants to believe in quick fixes. Having spent six years working for a weight-loss website, I get it—patience is a virtue, and it's a finite resource in most of us. While I firmly believe in the healing power of both major and minor mushrooms, please know that these mushrooms aren't magic. Some may have noticeable effects the first time you consume them, but most take a while. I felt calmer the first time I took a reishi tincture (an alcohol-based herbal medicine), for example, but I've never noticed any changes in my body from eating maitake or shiitake, other than not getting sick all winter (which could be attributed to any number of health-preserving measures I take). Just as you need to take an entire course of antibiotics, you also need to give holistic treatments time to take effect. How long and how much are questions you should discuss with your health care team.

No single herb, mushroom, or supplement is a cure-all. Don't expect major changes to happen overnight, and with any wellness or health regimen, you still have to put in the work. If you're taking cordyceps for stress but making no effort to reduce or manage the overwhelm you're experiencing, you can't expect your stress to simply disappear. As with herbs, supplements, or even pharmaceuticals, you need to do your part to deal with the root cause of your issues, not simply treat the symptoms.

Though Alan Muskat—who calls himself a "philosoforager, stand-up mycomedian, and epicure of the obscure"—has spent decades extolling the virtue of mushrooms, he is quick to caution that the intersection of mushroom cuisine and medicine does not yield a magic pill. Embracing mushrooms as part of a wellness routine should be part of changing your overall lifestyle.

"I make my own medicine, and I also take mushrooms as food," he says. "But I think the more important medicine is in the relationship that one establishes with the natural world."

I agree with Alan. Getting to know mushrooms—which herbs and spices complement which species, when they're "in season," and how they're best prepared—will connect you to nature, one bite and one meal at a time.

Shiitake
Lentinula edodes

Also known as: The oak mushroom (shiia is a Japanese oak)
Common uses: Immune health, cholesterol, antioxidant protection, skin health, liver support

The second most-consumed mushroom after button/cremini/portobellos, shiitake grows on fallen broadleaf trees across China, Japan, and other Asian countries with temperate climates, as well as in the U.S. It has been used as food and medicine for thousands of years in China and Japan.

Historically, shiitake was widely used as an immune booster in China and Japan, for everything from colds to cancer.[44] Studies have supported its antiviral and anti-cancer properties, and the lentinan it contains offers a boost for white blood cells and protects the immune system from oxidative stress. It can also lower cholesterol, protect your cells as you age, protect the liver (thereby also promoting healthy skin), and support the cardiovascular system. In TCM, it's considered to be strengthening and restorative.

Shiitake is the second most-studied mushroom after turkey tail. Official cancer research began in Japan in 1969, and shiitake has shown strong anti-tumor properties.

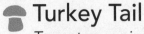 # Turkey Tail
Trametes versicolor

Also known as: *Coriolus versicolor; Polyporus versicolor*
Common uses: Immune health, cholesterol, liver support

I hadn't heard of turkey tail mushrooms until a couple of years ago, which surprised me because they are the best-researched mushroom. This mushroom—particularly the components PSP and PSK that are found in it—is a common cancer treatment in China and Japan. Turkey tail acts directly on tumors, preventing them from metastasizing.

Packed with antioxidants, turkey tails grow in overlapping clusters on fallen logs. The top is striped in shades of brown, white, gray, or blue, and the underside is white. They're commonly found in the U.S., Europe, and Asia.

Turkey tail has been used for its cholesterol-lowering abilities and immune-enhancing properties.[45] In TCM, it's used for treating infection, immune weakness, and inflammation in the upper respiratory, digestive, and urinary tracts.

Minor Medicinal Mushrooms

The mushrooms in this section tend to be prized more for their taste than their potential health benefits. As with all mushrooms, they contain beta-glucans so they support the immune system. While these mushrooms may not seem as impressive as the major ones, they're delicious and worth including in your diet.

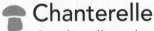 # Chanterelle
Cantharellus cibarius

Common uses: Immune health, detox

Their species name means "good to eat," and that is very true of chanterelles! These highly prized culinary mushrooms are found on the ground near conifers and broadleaf trees, and they range from bright orange to apricot in color. Chanterelles are native to Europe and North America. In TCM, they're used to tonify mucous membranes and help eyesight and the respiratory tract.

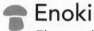 Enoki
Flammulina velutipes

Also known as: Winter mushrooms, snow peak mushrooms
Common uses: Immune health, beauty, antioxidant protection

Enoki is almost a major mushroom. Commonly consumed in Korea and Japan, enoki is white when cultivated due to lack of sunshine, and rusty brown when grown in nature. Enoki are said to help alleviate joint pain and inflammation, and they've been used to help the liver and ulcers.

Researchers did an epidemiological study of Japanese enoki farmers near the city of Nagano, where they noticed unusually low cancer rates compared to the general population. The primary difference was consumption of enoki.[47]

Enoki contain a cardiotoxic protein, according to Hobbs, so please cook them thoroughly as you would any mushroom.

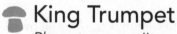 King Trumpet
Pleurotus eryngii

Also known as: French horn mushroom, king oyster mushroom
Common uses: Immune health, cholesterol

This large culinary mushroom with a thick white stem and small, flat brown cap is native to Europe, parts of Asia, the Middle East, and North Africa. It is commercially grown in Japan and the United States. King trumpet has been shown to lower cholesterol, triglyceride, and blood sugar levels in studies on rats.[48] It contains both ergothioneine and lovastatin.

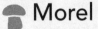 # Morel
Morchella esculenta

Common uses: Immune health, respiratory health

Found under poplars and pines, morel mushrooms seem to favor recently burned forests. Morels have immunosupportive qualities, but mostly these mushrooms are prized for their earthy taste.

In TCM, morels are used to treat excess phlegm and regulate qi, and they are a GI/stomach tonic too.

Raw or undercooked morels are toxic, so always cook them thoroughly and in a well-ventilated area.

 # Porcini/Bolete/Cèpe
Boletus edulis

Common uses: Immune health, heart health

These woodsy and leathery mushrooms are incredibly flavorful, yet they can't be cultivated. They're found under conifers and hardwoods in China, Europe, Russia, and North America.

Porcini, as they're best known in the U.S., are commonly consumed across Germany and Eastern Europe. Bohemian folklore says they were consumed to prevent cancer.

In TCM, they are used for leg and joint pain, in a traditional medicine called tendon-easing powder.[46]

 # White Button/Cremini/Portobello
Agaricus bisporus

Common uses: Immune health

Our plain old button mushrooms offer immune support, but they're often outshined by the more potent, exotic varieties of mushroom. In TCM, they're used as part of tendon-easing powder for joint and muscle pain, and they were used in Korea and China as a galact-agogue to increase breastmilk production.

Most button mushrooms (and cremini and portobellos) are commercially produced in Pennsylvania, specifically the small town of Kennett Square, where a group of Quakers in 1885 decided to fill some empty space in their greenhouses by growing mushrooms.[49] They hired Italian immigrants to work on their mushroom farms, and they, in turn, began their own crops. The portobello was discovered by accident when cremini mushrooms were allowed to grow longer. The rest is history. (Fun fact: The singular version is *cremino*.) Creminis, by the way, are baby bellos; they're simply young portobellos.

Button mushrooms contain the carcinogen agaritine, but you'd have to eat massive quantities every day for decades to do much damage. Still, Hobbs recommends eating them two to three times a week max, even when cooked.

Wood Ear
Auricularia spp auricula

Also known as: Tree ear, cloud ear, black fungus, mu erh
Common uses: GI tract support, cardiovascular health, skin

When my husband first encountered wood ears, he was skeptical that they were a mushroom. Once you see them, you'll understand why. This jelly fungus grows on trees like elder and spruce. It's semi-translucent and brown, and shaped like a cup or ear—frankly, they sometimes look like giant boogers. Highly prized in Japan, wood ear mushrooms grow across the U.S., Asia, and Europe. You've likely had them in hot and sour soup.

In TCM, they were used as a stomach tonic and to increase physical and mental energy.[50] In Europe, they were traditionally boiled and used for throat issues (per the Doctrine of Signatures) and applied topically to treat eye issues.

CHAPTER 3

Cooking with Mushrooms

One of my favorite annual events here in Asheville is the Medicines from the Earth Herb Symposium. There, I've spent entire days with Dr. Bove learning to make herbal salves, tinctures, and scrubs. I've sat through hours of lectures on adaptogenic herbs and the body's stress response system. And it was at Medicines where I first learned the science behind extracting mushrooms and cooking with them for medicinal purposes.

In 2016, ethnobotanist Marc Williams delivered a lecture on "Medicinal Mushrooms in the Kitchen and Apothecary." I furiously took notes as Marc gave a detailed overview of the mushrooms that now form the basis of my own mushroom *materia medica* (knowledge of healing ingredients). He shared chaga chai, turkey tail broth, and "bliss bites"—made with dried fruit, nuts, mushrooms, and spices. This workshop awakened me to a whole new set of ingredients. Until then, I was cooking with wild and cultivated mushrooms and using the local medicinal ones strictly as medicine. Marc's workshop—and, later, a team-building foraging excursion with him—inspired me to be more creative and integrate more medicinal mushrooms into my everyday diet, not just my herbal wellness protocol.

Since then, mushrooms have mushroomed in popularity. In Asheville, Dobra Tea serves sustainably sourced mushroom teas year-round. Fonta Flora, a microbrewery in nearby Morganton, released a limited-edition golden ale made with local chanterelles, cleverly named Ourcelium. And Villagers, a one-stop DIY shop for the crunchy, holistic-minded crowd, often can't keep their "Didn't It Rain" mushroom coffee blend in stock. The blend of chicory root, eleuthero root, dandelion root, burdock root, chaga, carob, orange peel, and cinnamon is good enough that you won't miss coffee, even on a chilly, rainy day.

This mushroom explosion comes at the perfect time. I don't think anyone would argue that our collective stress level seems to be on the rise, which in turn erodes our immune defenses. Mushrooms, take the wheel—we need your superpowers. Whether you're cooking up a mushroom frittata or whisking cordyceps into coffee, integrating mushrooms into your meals and drinks is a good way to get their benefits daily.

Cooking with mushrooms isn't difficult or particularly pricey. I add one or two fresh varieties to my shopping list weekly, and I buy a couple of powdered extracts at a time. Which mushrooms I choose depends on the season and my health—winter means more immune support, while summer means I might need energy and stamina.

My recipes strive to balance flavor and function, and I look to mushrooms for their umami as well as health support. You'll notice I rarely just add mushrooms to liquid (aside from broths). That's because it doesn't unlock their full flavor potential.

"You can't really beat the umami that you get from mushrooms in the plant-based food world, especially if you cook them right," says Nate Burrows, a photographer and sous chef at Plant, an award-winning vegan restaurant in Asheville. "If you don't brown your mushrooms, you're not really pulling out all the glutamate that's in them and not getting that deep earthy deliciousness

This chapter will teach you how to select, clean, store, and prepare mushrooms, from the common to the rare medicinal varieties.

Cooking with Mushrooms FAQs

Should I wash mushrooms?

Rinse fresh mushrooms lightly when they're dirty. If they're fairly clean, give them a wipe with a damp rag. Never soak cultivated mushrooms; they absorb too much water.

You can wash wild mushrooms that are particularly dirty (but always get a reliable identification before eating any wild mushrooms). Start by brushing off any visible dirt and debris, then quickly submerge them in water. Give them a swish and a final rinse, if needed, and dry them as quickly as possible. Reserve this treatment for only the dirtiest mushrooms, and then use high heat to dry out the mushrooms as quickly as possible.

How should I store mushrooms?

Store mushrooms in a paper bag (or, better yet for the environment, a cloth bag) to absorb excess moisture. Plastic doesn't allow mushrooms to "breathe," and you'll soon have slimy, smelly mushrooms. (If your mushrooms smell fishy, they've gone off and should be composted.) At home, you can store loose mushrooms in the produce drawer between layers of lint-free towels.

Should I look for conventional or organic mushrooms?

I prefer to eat only organic cultivated mushrooms (obviously wild ones can't be USDA Certified Organic). Conventional mushrooms ranked 34th on the Dirty Dozen list in 2017.[51]

Can I eat mushroom stems?

Softer stems are edible; those that are tough and fibrous like shiitakes' are not. Trim the ends of all stems with a paring knife. Reserve shiitake stems and slightly dried-out mushrooms for stocks.

What is the yield of a pound of fresh versus dried mushrooms?

One pound of fresh mushrooms yields about 3 ounces dried and about 5 to 6 cups sliced or chopped.

How can I integrate exotic mushrooms into my diet if I'm on a budget?

A little goes a long way when it comes to medicinal mushrooms. Mix them with common mushrooms to stretch their flavor. Buy a couple of ounces of healing mushrooms like shiitake or oyster and mix them with buttons or cremini.

When cooking with flavorful or more expensive mushrooms, slice them thinly to allow more of their flavor and nutrition to permeate the final dish.

How do I reconstitute dried mushrooms?

If you buy dried mushrooms from a supermarket, they'll likely be clean enough to simply soak in boiling water, drain (straining and reserving the soaking water if desired), and use. For wild mushrooms that are prone to debris, such as morels, you'll also need to give them a rinse.

In her book *Shroom*, Becky Selengut suggests using a clean French press to strain mushroom soaking liquid, and I've found this technique to be brilliant and simple.

Can I freeze mushrooms?

Yes, you can freeze mushrooms. As with most foods, freezing will interfere with quality, so keep that in mind. I froze some cooked lion's mane fillets as an experiment, and while the texture was softer and more watery than they had been fresh, they were still tasty. If you're concerned about bugs in wild mushrooms, freeze them for a few hours before preparing them.

Embracing the Flavor of Mushrooms

Can you embrace the healing power of mushrooms if you're not a fan of their flavor? I firmly believe you can train yourself to like new foods, especially those that are beneficial to you, and this cookbook contains plenty of recipes for mushroom skeptics or haters.

Let's start with the science behind picky eating. We are hard-wired not to trust bitter flavors, for example, as a way to suss out foods that are potentially toxic.[52] However, studies have repeatedly shown that if we keep trying, we can learn to like new foods, even those we initially dislike—mushrooms included.[53]

"Mushrooms have a very distinct flavor," concedes Skye Chilton, of the extracts company Real Mushrooms, so cooking with some healing mushrooms can be tough. We tend not to like the flavor of mushrooms straight-up, especially those that are bitter, like reishi. (Bitterness is indication of quality reishi, Chilton says, since the active triterpenes are bitter.)

However, bitter plays a crucial role in digestion, as we have receptors on the back of our tongue and throughout the GI tract that stimulate bile flow and the release of the digestive enzymes that help us break down food.

"So much of the modern diet is based on sweetness," Chilton says. Mushrooms are a good way to reintegrate bitter foods into your diet. Keep in mind as you try the recipes in this book that if you are a supertaster with a sensitive or highly refined palate, some of the dishes may have a, well, mushroomy aftertaste. Our Western palates are not accustomed to bitter or earthy flavors, so add more sweetener or salt as needed. Over time, you can reduce those masking flavors to allow the true flavor of each mushroom to shine through.

If it's the texture of mushrooms you dislike, take the advice of the Mushroom Council and blend them. Simply mince your mushrooms, then mix them into dishes as desired. The Council suggests combining minced mushrooms with ground meat to boost nutrition, save money, and reduce consumption of animal protein. While those are good tips, I suggest using ground or minced mushrooms on their own. Start with Basic Mushroom Duxelles (page 82).

How to Cook with Mushrooms

Simplicity is key when cooking with mushrooms. Burrows likes to press lightly seasoned mushrooms in a hot cast-iron skillet to maximize surface area. Muskat—who for two decades supplied rare mushrooms and foraged plants to some of the top restaurant in the South—says it doesn't take much at all for mushrooms to be delicious. A simple sauté with salt and pepper is his go-to treatment. Dr. Bove heeds the advice given to her by an expert forager she met in Vermont: sauté the mushrooms with butter and white wine, finish with good filtered water and parsley.

That's it. Though some of the recipes in this cookbook require more work, many of the savory dishes start with the concept of simplicity in mind. I often use alcohol when cooking mushrooms (I'll explain why later on page 47), along with a bit of neutral oil, salt, and pepper. I might add garlic or another allium at the end, but that's really all you need to do. When in doubt, especially when a mushroom is new to you, keep things simple to really allow the earthy deliciousness of the mushroom to shine.

Mushrooms are nature's sponges, and they will soak up as much flavor as you give them. Go easy on the marinade to start, or you may end up with overly salty or sweet mushrooms.

You've already learned my system for distinguishing between healing mushrooms (see page 22). Beyond major and minor mushrooms, there is another distinction that can help you quickly and easily know how to cook any edible mushroom you encounter: tough and tender.

The Tough and the Tender

There are two basic types of medicinal mushrooms: the culinary ones, meaning those that are soft and easily cooked, such as maitake, shiitake, and enoki; and the woody mushrooms that require a bit more coaxing to unlock their goodness, like reishi, chaga, and turkey tail. I like to call these the tough and the tender.

You don't see turkey tail risotto or stuffed reishi on restaurant menus. That's because no matter how long you cook those mushrooms, they'll always be too tough to chew. They also taste, well, medicinal. That's not to say they taste *bad*. I actually like the addition of these mushrooms in recipes. They just don't have the culinary appeal of a porcini or an oyster. Throughout the book, I use these tough mushrooms in broths and other slow-cooked recipes where their goodness can easily be imbibed. I also use them as powdered extracts in simpler dishes, from smoothies to kale chips.

THE TOUGH	THE TENDER
Chaga*	Button/Cremini/Portobello
Cordyceps*	Chanterelle
Reishi*	Enoki
Turkey Tail*	Lion's Mane*
	King Trumpet
	Maitake*
	Morel
	Oyster*
	Shiitake*
	Wood Ear

*Denotes major medicinal mushroom

Cooking Notes on Tender Mushrooms

Button/Cremini/Portobello

Flavor and texture: Mild but meaty, subtle flavor

- Holds shape after cooking; can be cooked a long time.

- Can be stuffed, sliced, or diced.

- Buttons should be purely white; dark brown spots indicate oxidation.

- Stems can be eaten (trim them slightly).

- Will keep 1 to 2 weeks in the fridge either in the original packaging or between layers of paper towels.

- When stuffing portobellos, trim the stem even with the bottom of the cap. Reserve stems for stock or dice them and add to sautés.

Burrows says we often miss the potential of the portobello by only cooking it once. He grills or broils it, then marinates it before roasting or sautéing. The toughness melts away, leaving you with a satisfying mouthfeel.

Chanterelle

Flavor and texture: Delicate texture; floral, sometimes sweet, buttery or peppery flavor; subtle apricot aroma

- Color ranges from pale white to bright yellow.

- Tear into strips instead of slicing; leave smaller caps whole.

- Simple preparations are best.

- Try sautéed and served with good bread, polenta, or whole grains.

- Should be firm, with no ragged edges.

- Store between layers of paper towels for up to 1 week.

Enoki

Flavor and texture: Delicate flavor and crunchy texture

- Should stand tall, not droop over.

- Add at the end of cooking; this is the exception to the "long, slow cooking" rule for mushrooms. But do cook thoroughly.

- Drying and freezing not recommended.

- Best in quick-cooking dishes.

- Store in the fridge for up to 1 week between layers of paper towels.

King Trumpet

Flavor and texture: Earthy flavor and meaty texture akin to seafood; stem resembles scallops when sliced

- Season and pair as you would seafood: white wine, capers, garlic, etc.

- Slice and score before marinating or searing.

- Use as you would oyster mushrooms.

- Avoid any mushrooms that are wrinkly. They should feel firm.

Lion's Mane

Flavor and texture: Like a cross between chicken and fish in both flavor and texture; mild and chewy, with a sweet scent

- Squeeze dry before searing or sautéing. Lion's mane are like sponges!

- Store in a paper bag or box to keep the "mane" intact.

- Will last up to 1 week in the fridge between layers of paper towels.

- Can be dried or cooked and frozen.

Maitake

Flavor and texture: Rich, meaty, yet delicate texture; very juicy; woodsy and sometimes yeasty or beerlike smell

- Trim the bottom of the stems, then slice or pull off the petals. Dice or mince the base of the stems.

- Though you usually shouldn't store mushrooms in plastic, the exception is the sealed, breathable packages that maitake and other mushrooms are sold in.

- They'll stay fresh up to a week, but if you only use half a package, store in a paper or cloth bag.

- Maximize their deep, woodsy flavor by searing and pressing.

- If you're buying them wild-harvested, avoid wet or brittle petals.

Morel

Flavor and texture: Rich and nutty; meaty

- Delicious sautéed or in cream sauces.

- Always cook them thoroughly in a well-ventilated area.

- Rinse or brush thoroughly to remove dirt from its signature pocked exterior

- One of the easiest mushrooms to identify, but always double-check. They have a distinctive cone shape that resembles a sponge.

- Dried morels are a good option and have a concentrated flavor.

- Should be firm and dry, with no wrinkles or sliminess.

- If not using stems, reserve for stocks.

- Store in the fridge for up to 1 week between layers of paper towels.

Oyster

Flavor and texture: Light and fruity taste; dense texture

- Incredibly easy to grow at home.

- Ranges in color from white to pale apricot and grayish blue.

- Add near the end; these don't need to cook a long time.

- Though you can chop them, I prefer to shred them or keep "petals" whole.

- I've been consistently less than impressed by supermarket oysters; grown them yourself or seek out a local grower.

- Flavor intensifies the longer they are cooked.

- Trim the caps near the stems, which you can reserve for stock.

- Stems are quite woody, so skip them in your sautés and other delicate dishes.

- Oysters should be slightly firm and crisp, with smooth tops (no wrinkles or dry edges).

- Store in the fridge for up to 1 week between layers of paper towels.

Porcini/Bolete/Cèpe

Flavor and texture: Luscious, meaty texture and nutty flavor

- Hearty and common in Italian cooking.

- Add to pasta sauces or risotto.

- Versatile and delicious—one of the most flavorful mushrooms I've encountered.

- Available frozen at Trader Joe's. Seek out fresh at farmers' markets.

Shiitake

Flavor and texture: Savory, rich, meaty, plentiful umami taste; dense and chewy texture, especially when broiled

- Among the earliest known sources of umami.

- Even meatier when dried and reconstituted.

- Slice them thinly, as their flavor can be quite strong.

- Reserve the stems for stock, or shred them finely and add to soups.

- Avoid shiitake with black spots or trim those away.

Wood Ear

Flavor and texture: Mild and slightly bitter; chewy yet firm when reconstituted or fresh

- One small packet will reconstitute to a full pound; usually a few pieces are enough for a dish.

- Their texture is more akin to sea vegetables than mushrooms.

- Dried wood ears will keep in a sealed container for up to 1 year.

- Chewy and mild, wood-ear mushrooms are a satisfying addition to any sauté or stir-fry.

- Thinly slice to highlight their texture.

- Available dried at Asian grocers and Whole Foods.

Powdered Dried Mushrooms versus Powdered Extracts

No matter the species you choose, you can't simply grind up dried mushrooms into a powder and toss them into your smoothie. The powders you see on store shelves and juice bar menus are actually powdered mushroom *extracts*, which are optimized for digestion and absorption. Some are extracted using only water, while others are dual-extracted using alcohol and water in a two-step process.

There are water-soluble and fat-soluble components in mushrooms; the former are best unlocked with a water decoction by simmering the mushrooms for 12 to 24 hours in water, while the latter are released through alcohol (by soaking the cooked mushrooms in alcohol for a few weeks). As a general rule, the immune compounds are water-soluble; the adaptogenic (hormone/stress) ones are alcohol-soluble.

In introductions and instructions, I sometimes use the phrase "mushrooms powders" for ease, but I am still referring to powdered mushroom extracts. To create powdered extracts, manufacturers dry the concentrated liquid extract, then finely grind the extract into a powder.

Most recipes call for servings of powdered extracts rather than specific measurements. Servings size will vary by brand; the mycelium-based powdered extracts tend to have larger by-volume servings than the fruiting body ones. (Mycelium-based extracts also have a milder taste, as the substrate mellows the intensity of the mushroom flavor.) Refer to your individual mushroom powders for more information.

Dual Extraction in the Kitchen

Dual extraction can even carry over to cooking with mushrooms. Many classic French and even some Chinese and Japanese dishes featuring mushrooms offer hints of this dual-extraction technique borrowed from medicine making. The mushrooms are sauteéd or stir-fried, then alcohol is used to deglaze the pan, and finally water, broth, or stock is added as the mushrooms slowly braise.

Cooking is an art; making extracts is an exact science. The recipes in this cookbook aim to maximize the benefits and flavor of mushrooms, but I did not test the beta-glucan or active constituent levels or protein digestibility of any dish.

Don't worry about the nitty-gritty science—leave that to the reputable brands who create mushroom extracts. Use this book as a way to foster a deeper appreciation of mushrooms and have a little fun with fungi! Together with the other whole foods and botanical superfoods in each recipe, these mushrooms can support your health as part of an overall nutritious diet.

Sourcing Quality Mushroom Products

In choosing mushroom extracts or tinctures, quality matters. Look for reputable brands, and shop at stores like your local co-op, Whole Foods, or other "healthy" supermarkets (like Sprouts or Earth Fare) that have their own set of standards for any products they carry. This will help you weed out the less reputable companies.

With mushrooms, there's a debate about whether products made from mycelium or fruiting bodies are better. In his 2017 *Herbalgram* article, Hobbs wrote, "Some researchers have found high levels of B[eta]-glucans in the fruiting bodies of tested species." However, he went on to say that more studies are needed to say for certain whether specific species show consistently higher levels of active constituents in mycelium versus fruiting bodies.

My personal opinion is that fruiting bodies are more concentrated, but there are also plenty of quality products made from mycelium.

Wild versus Cultivated Mushrooms

While I enjoy mushroom hunting, I'll admit that I could have made very few of the recipes in this book if I had relied solely on my hunter-gatherer skills. Like most of you, I buy my mushrooms at the supermarket and farmers' market. This allows me the peace of mind that I'm consuming only verified species of mushrooms that have been grown in clean, unpolluted environments. Foraging for your own mushrooms is certainly a fun adventure, but you can still reap the benefits of mushrooms if you, like me, rely on cultivated ones.

According to Hobbs, in tests, wild mushrooms have been shown to be more nutritious than cultivated in many cases, but cultivated mushrooms from reputable sources are still quite nutritious.[54] This just goes to show that nature knows best, but skilled farmers know plenty.

Wild mushrooms are an affordable option—outside is free!—but always seek the input of a mushroom expert before eating anything you've foraged. Each wild mushroom has a season, which enthusiasts know well. Morels are a harbinger of spring, while chanterelles and reishi are plentiful in summer, for example.

Cultivated mushrooms are available year-round. Mushroom farms don't resemble vegetable farms. They're grown indoors in sterile production facilities. It wasn't so long ago—a few decades—that the white button mushroom might have been the only variety available in your local supermarket. Thankfully for mycophiles, medicinal varieties like oysters and maitake are now widely cultivated, and at-home grow kits allow you to cultivate reishi, lion's mane, and even turkey tail indoors with very little effort. You can also inoculate certain types of logs with mushroom spores and grow others, like shiitake, outdoors. Not all mushrooms can be cultivated. Certain varieties, including truffles, have notoriously resisted all efforts at cultivation.

The more exotic varieties of cultivated mushrooms mostly come from California, though you can likely find someone in your area growing mushrooms.

If you want to get into foraging, find someone in your area to teach you. There is no substitute for the one-on-one (or small group) teacher-student experience. Since the risk of misidentifying a mushroom for an inedible or toxic variety is high, work with someone like Alan Muskat or Abby Artemisia who knows that they're doing. This is also a great way to keep traditional storytelling and folklore alive. It wasn't until I moved to the mountains than I realized how valuable the connection to nature is. Sure, I hiked and admired scenery, but living in a temperate rainforest, where you might encounter a bear or a patch of wild blueberries (or both!), makes you appreciate traditional skills like wildcrafting, foraging, and the like. I trust myself to identify only a few mushrooms in nature: morels, chanterelles, reishi, and lion's mane. However, even after years of experience, I err on the side of being overly cautious. I'm usually a "look but don't pick" mushroom enthusiast.

What's cool about mushrooms is that they can seemingly make something from nothing. They appear as if by magic, from spores invisible to the naked eye. And they can grow spectacularly on scraps. While in life, it is usually true that you get out what you put in, with mushrooms, you reap far more than what you sow!

Dried versus Fresh Mushrooms

Drying prolongs the shelf life of mushrooms. Wild mushrooms have shorter life spans once picked, and some, such as porcini, spoil so quickly that you'll usually find them dried. You need to extract mushrooms to unlock their medicinal qualities, of which there are many. That's why most of the recipes in this book call for powdered mushroom extract versus ground mushrooms.

CHAPTER 4

———— ✕ ————

Breakfast

Start your day off right, with nutritious and delicious breakfasts featuring mushrooms. In this chapter, you'll learn how to start integrating mushroom powders (powdered extracts, that is) into your meals. You'll find a balance of sweet and savory dishes, whether you're craving a leisurely weekend brunch or a quick weekday meal.

Orange-Cardamom Oatmeal

Warm and comforting, oatmeal is rich in soluble fiber, the type that becomes a thick gel when combined with water. Soluble fiber helps stabilize blood sugar levels and lower cholesterol. Oats are also soothing for the digestive system. I've added orange and cardamom not only for flavor but for digestive support too. Walnuts add a boost of protein and omega-3s, as well as crunch.

During their early stages of growth, oats are also used to support the nervous system—think of them like an oatmeal bath for your nerves. Harvested when their tender tops are milky, young oats are a nervine and classic tonic, often used with adaptogens for stress.

SERVES: 4 | PREP AND COOK TIME: 15 minutes

2 cups old-fashioned oats

4 servings powdered mushroom extract

½ cup raisins

½ teaspoon ground cardamom

2 tablespoons orange zest

juice of 1 orange

¼ cup maple syrup (optional)

½ cup chopped walnuts

1. Prepare the oats according to package directions, adding water to achieve the desired consistency.

2. Stir in the remaining ingredients except for the walnuts. Divide the oatmeal into four bowls, then top with the walnuts. Serve immediately.

✚ Digestion, Immune

Savory Mushroom Oatmeal

If you've never tried savory oatmeal, you're missing out. Like polenta, congee, or grits, oatmeal can be a neutral canvas for any ingredients you like, sweet or savory. I prefer the savory route, especially mushrooms, onions, and celery sautéed with herbes de Provence. I serve this for breakfast throughout the year, changing up the herbs with the seasons.

SERVES: 1 or 2 | PREP AND COOK TIME: 15 minutes

1 tablespoon neutral oil or ghee

½ cup sliced mushrooms (maitake, button, shiitake, porcini, and/or cremini)

¼ cup diced onions

1 stalk celery, diced

½ teaspoon herbes de Provence or poultry seasoning

1 cup old-fashioned oats

1 cup mushroom broth or water

1 cup greens, such as chopped kale or spinach

2 tablespoons nutritional yeast, plus more to top

salt and pepper, to taste

1. Place a large saucepan over medium-high heat. Add the oil or ghee, then the mushrooms, onions, celery, and herbes de Provence or poultry seasoning. Cook, stirring often, for about 5 minutes, until the vegetables start to get some color.

2. Stir in the oats and the broth or water. Heat until simmering, then reduce the heat to medium-low, stirring often, until the oats are thick and creamy, about 5 minutes. Stir in the remaining ingredients, seasoning to taste with salt and pepper.

3. Serve immediately, garnished as desired with more nutritional yeast.

✚
Immune

Loaded Mushroom-Avocado Sweet Potato Toast

I prefer savory to sweet, especially first thing in the morning. Avocado toast—along with savory oats like those on page 53—is on my menu a few times a week. Over the years, I've perfected mine for (what I believe) to be optimal morning nutrition: I start with a thick slice of sweet potato; add fermented veggies like kimchi or sauerkraut for gut health; nutritional yeast for B vitamins, fiber, and protein; and sautéed mushrooms for immune support. I top it with sprouts for their intense phytonutrients, a smattering of chives or scallions for flavor, and sesame or hemp seeds for crunch and a final boost of nutrition.

SERVES: 1 | PREP AND COOK TIME: 15 minutes

2 (¾-inch) slices from a large sweet potato, peeled if desired

1 clove garlic

½ avocado, mashed

½ cup Basic Sautéed Mushrooms (page 68)

2 tablespoons prepared kimchi or sauerkraut

2 tablespoons nutritional yeast

2 tablespoons sprouts

1 tablespoon snipped chives or sliced scallions

1 tablespoon toasted sesame seeds or hemp hearts

1. Toast the sweet potatoes as desired. I use a toaster oven and toast for two full cycles so they're nice and tender.

2. Rub the garlic clove over the toasted sweet potato. Top with the avocado, then the mushrooms, kimchi or sauerkraut, nutritional yeast, sprouts, chives or scallions, and sesame seeds or hemp hearts. Serve immediately.

Immune

Matcha Bowl with Lion's Mane

Strapped for time in the morning? Combine caffeine and breakfast in this matcha smoothie bowl. Lion's mane gives it a memory-boosting effect, making this a go-to breakfast anytime you have a major presentation or test. To help you reach your quota of veggies for the day, I sneak in some greens. If you prefer to drink your smoothie, add more liquid, and serve in a jar or glass.

To keep recipes simple, I usually list "milk" in the ingredients list. Unless specified, it's up to you whether you choose cow's milk or a non-dairy version. My default milk choice is plain, unsweetened soy milk.

SERVES: 1 | PREP TIME: 10 minutes

For the bowl:

1 frozen banana

½ cup frozen pineapple chunks

½ cup milk

1 scoop vanilla protein powder

1 to 2 cups spinach or kale

1 serving powdered lion's mane extract

1 ½ teaspoons matcha powder

For the topping:

hemp hearts

blueberries

ground flaxseed

Combine the ingredients for the bowl in a blender until smooth. Use a tamper to push down the ingredients as needed (to avoid needing extra liquid). Transfer the smoothie to a bowl, then garnish with toppings as desired.

✚ Energy, Immune, Memory, Nervous System

Poached Soft Tofu or Eggs in Mushroom Broth

Starting the day with a warm soup sounds so comforting, especially in winter or after a chilly a.m. workout, so I decided to create my own morning mushroom soup. With a miso-mushroom base, it's particularly delightful when you're fighting a cold or on the mend.

SERVES: 4 | PREP AND COOK TIME: 25 minutes

1 quart (4 cups) mushroom broth

2 cups water

4 scallions, whites and greens, thinly sliced

1 bunch kale, leaves only, thinly sliced

1 cup tender mushrooms, thinly sliced

¼ teaspoon black pepper

4 eggs or 1 pound soft tofu

¼ cup white miso paste

2 cups prepared brown rice

1. Place the mushroom broth in a 2-quart saucepan. Add the water and bring to a boil over high heat. Stir in the scallions, kale, mushrooms, and pepper. Reduce heat so it's barely simmering.

2. If using eggs, crack one into a small dish. Swirl the simmering broth, then slide the egg gently into the center of the pan. Cook for 4 minutes, then transfer to a serving bowl. Repeat with the remaining eggs. If using tofu, add the tofu to the broth and cook until heated through, about 5 minutes.

3. Transfer 1 cup of the broth to a small bowl, and whisk in the miso paste. Stir the miso mixture into the broth.

4. Divide the rice into four bowls, then top with one quarter of the broth, plus one egg or one quarter of the tofu, and one quarter of the vegetables.

✚
Immune

Sweet Potato-Mushroom Hash

Sometimes I like to play a game at breakfast: How many servings of vegetables can I possibly squeeze into one meal? With nearly the whole rainbow on one plate, this generously spiced hash might set a record, yet it only takes 30 minutes to make. The vibrant colors make me feel like I'm really treating my body right.

SERVES: 4 | PREP AND COOK TIME: 30 minutes

2 tablespoons safflower oil

2 cups diced tender mushrooms

1 large yellow onion, diced

1 teaspoon ground cumin

¼ teaspoon dried thyme

¼ teaspoon smoked paprika

⅛ teaspoon black pepper, plus more to taste

1 medium red or yellow bell pepper, diced

2 large sweet potatoes, finely diced or shredded

3 cloves garlic, minced

4 cups baby spinach

¼ cup nutritional yeast

2 tablespoons toasted sesame seeds

salt, to taste

1. Place a large, deep skillet over medium-high heat. Add the oil, then add the mushrooms and onion. Cook, stirring often, for about 5 minutes, until they start to soften and get some color.

2. Lower the heat to medium, then add the cumin, thyme, paprika, and pepper. Cook another minute, then add the bell pepper and sweet potato. Cover and cook for 5 minutes, stirring occasionally.

3. Uncover, add the garlic, and cook another 8 to 10 minutes, until the vegetables are tender but not mushy. Remove from the heat and stir in the spinach. Season to taste with salt and pepper, and stir in the nutritional yeast. Serve immediately, topped with the sesame seeds.

✚ Immune

Cauliflower-Mushroom Scramble

Packed with antioxidants and natural detoxifiers, this scramble is perfect for a morning after you overindulge. Cruciferous vegetables like cauliflower and kale, as well as turmeric, promote liver detoxification. Enoki, maitake, and shiitake also support the liver, making this brunch a good choice after a wild night out. Pair it with a Shiitake Bloody Mary (page 241) if you must.

SERVES: 4 | PREP AND COOK TIME: 30 minutes

2 tablespoons safflower oil

1 cup mushrooms, such as enoki, shiitake, and/or maitake

1 small yellow onion, diced

1 medium red or yellow bell pepper, diced

1 teaspoon ground cumin

1 teaspoon yellow curry powder

½ teaspoon ground turmeric

¼ teaspoon dried thyme

¼ teaspoon smoked paprika

⅛ teaspoon black pepper, plus more to taste

pinch of cayenne pepper (optional)

3 cloves garlic, minced

6 cups cauliflower rice, fresh or frozen

1 bunch kale, leaves only, shredded

8 eggs or 1 pound firm tofu, crumbled

1 teaspoon tamari

salt, to taste

1. Place a large, deep skillet over medium-high heat. Add the oil, then add the mushrooms, onion, and bell pepper. Cook, stirring often, for about 5 minutes, until they start to soften and get some color.

2. Lower the heat to medium, then add the cumin, curry powder, turmeric, thyme, smoked paprika, black pepper, and cayenne pepper, if using. Cook another minute, then add the garlic and cauliflower. Cover and cook for five minutes, stirring occasionally.

3. Uncover, add the kale, and cook another 5 to 7 minutes, until the vegetables are tender but not mushy. Add the eggs or tofu, and stir to combine. Cook, stirring often, until the eggs are cooked or the tofu

is warm, about 5 minutes. Season to taste with salt and black pepper, and serve immediately.

✚ Beauty, Detox, Immune, Liver

Rosemary-Chanterelle Scramble

Chanterelles are right at home in a scramble. With rosemary, chives, and plenty of mushrooms, this dish is worthy of weekend brunch, but it's fast enough for a weekday. It's equally delicious with soft tofu or eggs.

SERVES: 4 | PREP AND COOK TIME: 15 minutes

2 cups fresh chanterelle mushrooms or 2 ounces dried chanterelles

8 eggs or 1 pound soft tofu

2 tablespoons milk (optional)

1 tablespoon safflower oil

1 tablespoon butter

1 tablespoon minced fresh rosemary

1 clove garlic, minced

¼ cup snipped chives

toast, for serving (optional)

salt and pepper, to taste

1. If using dried chanterelles, soak them in hot water for at least 30 minutes, then drain. Chop the mushrooms.

2. Whisk the eggs with the milk (skip if using tofu), seasoning with salt and pepper. If using tofu, break into chunks and season with salt and pepper.

3. Place a large nonstick skillet over medium heat. Add the safflower oil and butter. Once the butter has melted, add the mushrooms, rosemary, salt, and pepper. Cook for about 5 minutes, until the mushrooms are soft and fragrant. Add the garlic, chives, and the eggs or tofu. Cook, stirring often, until the eggs are set or the tofu is heated through, about 5 minutes.

4. Serve immediately, with toast if desired.

✚ Cardiovascular, Detox, Immune

Slow Cooker Shiitake-Scallion Congee

Congee is simple comfort food, and this easy-to-digest Chinese rice porridge is perfect on cold winter mornings and after times when the belly is off. If you have a slow cooker with a sauté setting, it streamlines the process. Though I call for shiitakes here to promote natural detoxification, you can use any tender mushroom, and can even add tough ones to the slow cooker.

SERVES: 4 | PREP AND COOK TIME: 8 hours, 10 minutes

1 teaspoon sesame oil

4 shiitake mushroom caps, thinly sliced

1 medium shallot, minced

2 teaspoons grated fresh ginger

4 cloves garlic, minced

1 tablespoon tamari

1 cup long-grain brown rice

2 cups mushroom broth

6 cups water

For serving:

sliced scallions

miso paste

sriracha or chili sauce

toasted sesame seeds

toasted sesame oil

salt

1. Heat the sesame oil in a slow cooker using the sauté setting (or in a saucepan over medium-high heat). Add the shiitakes and shallot. Cook, stirring often, for about 5 minutes, until the mushrooms are darkened and fragrant. Add the ginger and garlic, and cook another minute.

2. Turn off the sauté setting. If cooking on the stove, transfer the mushrooms and shallots to a slow cooker. Add the tamari, rice, broth, and water.

3. Set slow cooker to low heat for 8 hours. When finished, the mixture should be cloudy and slightly thick, and the rice soft.

4. Scoop into four bowls and add garnishes as desired. If you're skipping the miso, you likely will need to add salt.

✚ Beauty, Detox, Immune

Maitake "Bacon"–Avocado Sandwiches

This BLT is a cardiologist's dream—we use maitake "bacon" in place of the real deal, add avocado in place of mayo, and swap sprouts for lettuce. Mushrooms are quite convincing as a bacon swap. The bacon flavor comes from a salty, smoky, slightly sweet marinade, and using a cast-iron skillet gets the crispy edges you crave.

SERVES: 4 | PREP AND COOK TIME: 2 hours, 30 minutes

For the maitake bacon:

2 tablespoons safflower oil

1 tablespoon maple syrup

1 tablespoon red miso paste

½ teaspoon black pepper

½ teaspoon smoked paprika

1 clove garlic, minced

⅛ teaspoon liquid smoke

¼ teaspoon cayenne pepper (optional)

1 tablespoon nutritional yeast

1 bunch maitake mushrooms, petals separated

For the sandwich:

8 slices whole-grain or sourdough bread

2 ripe avocados, pitted and mashed

½ cup nutritional yeast

1 medium ripe tomato, sliced

½ cup prepared kimchi or sauerkraut

½ cup sprouts (alfalfa, broccoli, etc.)

1. To prepare the maitake bacon, combine all the ingredients except for the maitake in a shallow dish with a lid. Add the maitake, toss to coat, cover the dish, and marinate in the refrigerator for at least 2 hours or up to overnight.

2. When ready to eat, place a large, well-seasoned cast-iron skillet over medium-high heat and line a baking sheet with parchment paper. Once the skillet is hot, add the mushrooms in a single layer, draining off any liquid. Cook, stirring occasionally, for 5 to 6 minutes, until the mushrooms are crispy and dark around the edges.

3. Remove the mushrooms from the heat and transfer to a parchment-lined baking sheet.

4. Toast the bread to your desired doneness. Top with the maitake bacon and remaining ingredients.

✚
Blood Sugar, Immune

Why Mushroom Bacon Matters

"Yes, bacon really is killing us," proclaimed a March 2018 article in *The Guardian*.[55] The World Health Organization has classified processed meats like bacon as a group 1 carcinogen, meaning there is sufficient evidence to show they cause cancer, especially that of the colon.[56]

Using fiber-rich mushrooms in place of processed meats allows you to keep the sweet, salty, smokiness you crave, without putting your health at risk.

Chaga Acai Bowl

Take one look at acai, and you know it is bursting with antioxidants. Native to South America, this dark purple fruit has a unique, complex flavor—somewhat like a not-so-sweet raspberry with a hint of very dark chocolate. I like to sweeten it naturally with a ripe banana, then add even more antioxidants with pomegranate juice, frozen berries, and chaga, plus beet and ginger powders.

SERVES: 1 or 2 | PREP TIME: 10 minutes

1 banana

½ cup pomegranate juice

½ cup water

1 cup frozen berries

2 packets frozen acai

1 scoop protein powder (optional)

1 tablespoon beet powder

1 teaspoon grated fresh ginger

1 serving powdered chaga extract

For serving:

nuts

seeds

bee pollen

fresh berries

coconut flakes

1. Combine all the ingredients except garnishes in a blender, using a tamper to help blend the fruit without using extra liquid.

2. Transfer to a bowl and garnish as desired.

✚
Antioxidant, Immune

Chanterelle Toast with Ricotta

Ricotta is a cheese that's quite high in protein, and it's subtly sweet, which pairs well with the sweet nuttiness of chanterelles. (Kite Hill's almond milk ricotta is a tasty dairy-free option.) This simple yet elegant toast comes together in just 10 minutes.

SERVES: 1 or 2 | PREP TIME: 10 minutes

1 tablespoon butter or olive oil

1 small shallot, minced

½ teaspoon minced fresh rosemary

4 chanterelle mushrooms, wiped clean and chopped

¼ cup almond or whole milk ricotta

2 slices sourdough bread, toasted

salt and pepper, to taste

1. Place a small skillet over medium-high heat. Add the butter or oil to the hot pan, then add the shallot and rosemary. Sauté for about 3 minutes, until the shallot starts to soften and get some color. Add the chanterelles and cook another 5 minutes. Season with salt and pepper.

2. Spread the ricotta on the slices of toast. Top with the chanterelle mixture. Serve immediately.

✚ Cardiovascular, Detox, Immune

Apple-Cinnamon Chaga Waffles

Chaga blends right into these well-spiced apple-cinnamon waffles. If you, like me, prefer things to be less sweet, choose a tart apple. Cinnamon not only helps keep your blood sugar in check, it also lends a natural sweetness. These can be made in bulk and frozen.

SERVES: 4 | PREP AND COOK TIME: 30 minutes

1 cup whole-wheat pastry flour

2 tablespoons ground flaxseed

3 servings powdered chaga extract

1 ½ teaspoons baking powder

½ teaspoon ground cinnamon

⅛ teaspoon salt

1 medium apple, diced

1 cup milk

1 tablespoon safflower oil

1 tablespoon maple syrup, plus more for serving

½ teaspoon vanilla extract

butter, for serving (optional)

1. Preheat a waffle iron.

2. In a medium bowl, stir together the flour, flaxseed, chaga extract, baking powder, cinnamon, and salt until well-combined. Toss the apples with the dry ingredients.

3. Combine the milk, oil, the tablespoon of maple syrup, and vanilla in a small bowl, then pour into the dry ingredients, stirring until just combined.

4. Grease the waffle iron, then scoop a heaping half-cup of batter into the hot waffle iron. Cook for 6 to 7 minutes, or until cooked through. Repeat with remaining batter.

5. Serve immediately, with maple syrup and butter, if desired.

✚ Antioxidant, Immune

CHAPTER 5

Appetizers and Sides

Mushrooms find their way into my meals daily, sometimes in multiple courses of the same meal. If you're warming up to the idea of giving mushrooms a place in your regular meal rotation, start with an appetizer or side. This chapter uses tender mushrooms that will be mostly familiar to you, including white button and cremini, in both expected and innovative ways.

For you mushroom lovers, there are plenty of exotic mushrooms, too: enoki, shiitake, maitake, and lion's mane among them.

You'll notice that many recipes call simply call for "tender mushrooms," giving you the freedom to choose your favorite or what's in season.

Basic Sautéed Mushrooms

This is the basic cooking method I use for sautéing any tender mushroom. Use these mushrooms as a simple side, mix them into whole grains, or make a roux and add broth to create a pan sauce or gravy.

SERVES: 4 to 6 | PREP AND COOK TIME: 30 minutes

1 tablespoon safflower oil

4 cups tender mushrooms, sliced

½ teaspoon dried herbs of choice

1 medium shallot or ½ small yellow onion, diced

⅛ teaspoon black pepper, plus more to taste

2 tablespoons dry sherry or ¼ cup dry white wine

salt, to taste

1. Place a large skillet over medium-high heat. Add the oil, and once warm, add the mushrooms, herbs, and shallot or onion, along with the pepper and a pinch of salt. Cook, stirring often, for about 5 minutes, until the mixture starts to soften and get some color.

2. Lower the heat to medium. Add the sherry or wine, then scrape the bottom of the pan to release any brown bits. Cook for 2 minutes more to allow the alcohol to evaporate.

3. Remove from heat, season with more salt and pepper to taste, and serve immediately.

✚
Immune

Lion's Mane "Crab Cake" Patties

These patties highlight the exquisite flavor of lion's mane. This mushroom truly does taste like seafood or chicken, with a satisfyingly similar texture. Here, generous "lumps" of lion's mane are paired with red bell pepper, scallions, and capers in a light yet filling patty reminiscent of crab cakes.

SERVES: 4 to 6 | PREP AND COOK TIME: 30 minutes

¼ cup mushroom broth

1 teaspoon Dijon mustard

½ cup soft tofu

1 tablespoon extra-virgin olive oil

2 tablespoons lemon juice

2 cup lion's mane mushrooms, pulled into bite-size pieces and excess water removed

1 medium red bell pepper, diced

1 scallion, white and green parts, thinly sliced

1 tablespoon capers

½ cup whole wheat pastry flour

½ teaspoon salt

⅛ teaspoon black pepper

1. Preheat the oven to 425°F. Line a baking sheet with parchment paper.

2. Blend the broth, mustard, tofu, olive oil, and lemon juice together in a mini food processor or blender. Set aside.

3. In a large bowl, toss the lion's mane with the bell pepper, scallions, and capers. Mix in the flour, salt, and pepper. Add the tofu mixture, stirring until just combined. Wet your hands, then form the mixture into 4 to 6 patties. Place the patties on the prepared baking sheet, flattening them to be about ¾ inch thick.

4. Bake for 15 minutes, then flip and bake another 20 minutes, until golden brown and cooked through. If you desire more color and a crispier exterior, pan fry in a small amount of oil before serving.

✚ Immune, Memory, Nervous System

Warm Potato Salad with Morels and Pecan-Herb Dressing

Morels need very little; their deliciousness exceeds even the humblest of preparations. This spring potato salad highlights the smoky earthiness of morels. Use the smallest new potatoes and the freshest herbs for a simple yet satisfying salad.

SERVES: 4 to 6 | PREP AND COOK TIME: 30 minutes

2 pounds red new potatoes, halved or quartered

1 cup mushroom broth

few sprigs fresh thyme, dill, or tarragon

1 cup water

2 tablespoons safflower oil

½ pound fresh morels, large ones halved

salt and pepper, to taste

For the dressing:

2 tablespoons minced red onion or 1 small shallot, minced

2 tablespoons minced flat-leaf parsley

½ teaspoon fresh thyme leaves

1 teaspoon minced fresh tarragon

1 teaspoon minced fresh dill

2 tablespoons lemon juice

2 tablespoons white wine vinegar

1 teaspoon Dijon mustard

¼ cup extra-virgin olive oil

1. Place the potatoes in a large pot with a lid. Add the broth and herbs, water, and a generous amount of salt and pepper. Bring to a boil over high heat, reduce the heat to medium, and simmer for 15 to 20 minutes, stirring often, until the potatoes are tender. Most of the water and broth will evaporate. If more liquid is needed before the potatoes are cooked, add ½ cup of water.

2. Meanwhile, make the dressing. In a jar with a lid, combine the onion or shallot, parsley, thyme, tarragon, dill, lemon juice, vinegar, and mustard. Shake to combine, then add the olive oil and shake again.

3. Heat the safflower oil in a medium skillet over medium-high heat. Add the morels, and season generously with salt and pepper. Cook for about 5 minutes, until the mushrooms start to soften and darken. Reduce the heat to medium and cook for 5 minutes more.

4. Toss the potatoes and any leftover cooking liquid with the morels and their cooking liquid. Add the dressing, toss to combine, and serve immediately.

✚
Immune

Enoki-Scallion Chickpea Fritters

Delicate enoki make perfect pakoras, the spiced Indian fritters coated in high-protein chickpea batter. Traditionally deep fried, these fritters are pan-fried to keep them light and fluffy. You can swap in any herb blend for the garam masala and turmeric; try Old Bay, Italian spices, or smoked paprika and cumin.

SERVES: 4 to 6 | PREP AND COOK TIME: 30 minutes

For the batter:

½ cup chickpea flour

1½ teaspoons garam masala

½ teaspoon baking powder

¼ teaspoon ground turmeric

½ teaspoon salt

½ cup mushroom broth

¼ cup water

For the fritters:

1 bunch enoki mushrooms, ends trimmed, mostly separated and cut into thirds

2 scallions, white and green parts, thinly sliced

2 tablespoons safflower oil, divided

salt, for sprinkling

1. In a medium bowl, combine all the ingredients for the batter. It should be slightly thin.

2. Fold the enoki and scallions into the batter.

3. Line a baking sheet with paper towels. Place a large nonstick skillet over medium-high heat. Warm 1 tablespoon of the safflower oil, then scoop ¼ cup portions of the enoki batter into the pan, leaving space between each one.

4. Cook for 2 minutes per side, or until evenly browned and cooked through. Place on the prepared baking sheet. Add the remaining oil as needed, and repeat with the rest of the batter. Before serving, reheat all the fritters in the skillet if necessary, and sprinkle with salt.

✚ Beauty, Immune

Italian Celery–Mushroom Salad

The classic Italian version of this salad uses raw mushrooms. In addition to committing one of my cardinal sins of mushrooms (never eat them raw), there wasn't enough textural contrast for my liking. Sautéing the mushrooms then adding them to a lightly dressed salad of cool, crisp celery and parsley creates a more pleasurable final dish.

SERVES: 4 to 6 | PREP AND COOK TIME: 30 minutes

For the salad:

- 1 tablespoon white wine vinegar
- 2 tablespoons lemon juice
- 1 teaspoon lemon zest
- ¼ teaspoon black pepper
- ¼ teaspoon salt
- 2 tablespoons extra virgin olive oil
- 1 bunch celery, including the leaves and small stalks, thinly sliced
- ¼ cup flat-leaf parsley leaves, roughly chopped

For the mushrooms:

- 1 tablespoon olive oil
- 2 cup sliced tender mushrooms
- 2 cloves garlic, minced
- salt and pepper, to taste

1. Prepare the dressing by whisking together the vinegar, lemon juice, lemon zest, pepper, salt, and olive oil in a medium bowl. Add the celery and parsley, and toss to combine. Refrigerate while you prepare the mushrooms.

2. Place a medium skillet over medium heat. Add the olive oil, then the mushrooms and garlic. Season with salt and pepper, and cook for about 10 minutes, until tender and starting to darken, stirring occasionally.

3. Either toss the hot mushrooms with the celery salad and serve immediately, or let cool completely, then toss with the rest of the salad.

✚ Immune

Enoki Bundles

Strips of marinated yuba (tofu sheets) hold together small bunches of enoki for a quick appetizer that highlights these tender mushrooms. Quickly pan-fried and doused in a sweet, tangy marinade, these bundles are fun finger food. If desired, you can also just sear the mushrooms and skip the yuba.

SERVES: 4 to 6 | PREP AND COOK TIME: 1 hour, 30 minutes

For the marinade:

¼ cup rice wine vinegar

3 tablespoons soy sauce or tamari

2 tablespoons sugar

1 tablespoon toasted sesame oil

For the bundles:

2 sheets fresh yuba (tofu skins)

1 bunch enoki mushrooms, ends trimmed, divided into 12 equal-size bundles

1 tablespoon safflower oil

2 scallions, white and green parts, thinly sliced, for garnish

1. Combine the marinade ingredients in a shallow dish with a lid. Dredge the yuba in the marinade and refrigerate for 1 hour.

2. After an hour, remove the yuba, reserving the marinade. Trim each sheet into six long strips.

3. Carefully but tightly roll one strip of yuba around each bunch of enoki, leaving both ends visible.

4. Heat the safflower oil in a large skillet over medium-high heat. Add the enoki bundles, leaving plenty of room between them. Cook for 1 minute, then flip and cook 1 minute more. Add the reserved marinade, cover, and cook for 1 more minute.

5. Remove from the heat and serve immediately, garnished with the scallions.

✚ Beauty, Immune

Simple Braised Cabbage and Mushrooms

This hearty side is simple and satisfying, perfect for a winter supper. With warming caraway—a digestive aid that can ease gas and bloating—this dish can help lighten up any meal. Serve alongside rich pastas and stews. Cabbage and onions are also both immune boosters, so keep this dish on weekly rotation all through the colder months. If you are dairy-free, feel free to swap in vegan "butter" or oil in this dish or any in the book. I tested my recipes with Earth Balance and homemade vegan butter.

SERVES: 4 to 6 | PREP AND COOK TIME: 1 hour, 15 minutes

1 tablespoon safflower oil

2 cups tender mushrooms, thinly sliced

1 large yellow onion, thinly sliced

1 small head green cabbage, cored and thinly sliced

1 teaspoon caraway seeds

1 teaspoon celery seeds

½ teaspoon salt

¼ teaspoon black pepper

3 tablespoons butter

1 cup mushroom broth

1. Preheat the oven to 425°F.

2. Coat a 9 x 11-inch baking dish with the safflower oil. Layer in the mushrooms, onion, and cabbage. Sprinkle on the caraway and celery seeds, season with salt and pepper, and dot with the butter and broth.

3. Cover the dish with a sheet of parchment paper and an inverted baking sheet.

4. Bake for 30 minutes, stir, and bake for another 30 minutes. Remove the baking sheet, stir again, and bake another 15 minutes, uncovered, until tender and starting to brown on the top and sides. Serve immediately.

✚ Immune

Enoki Veggie Rolls with Spirulina Quinoa

Enoki adds great texture to sushi-style rolls. Protein-rich quinoa stands in for rice, and cooling, detoxifying spirulina—a single-cell blue-green algae—adds an oceanlike flavor as well as numerous nutrients. Cucumber, avocado, and scallions further boost the beauty appeal of these rolls. You can find spirulina in the supplements aisle of most co-ops and larger grocery stores. Swap in 1 or 2 spirulina or chlorella (a green algae) tablets if you can't find the powder.

SERVES: 4 to 6 | PREP AND COOK TIME: 45 minutes

For the quinoa:

⅓ cup quinoa

1 teaspoon spirulina powder

1 teaspoon toasted sesame oil

¼ teaspoon salt

1 tablespoon chia seeds

For the enoki:

1 teaspoon toasted sesame oil

1 teaspoon grated fresh ginger

1 teaspoon tamari

1 tablespoon maple syrup

4 (1-inch) bundles enoki mushrooms

To assemble:

4 sheets nori

1 avocado, sliced

½ small English cucumber, sliced lengthwise into 8 pieces

4 scallions

1. Prepare the quinoa according to package directions. Once cooked, remove from heat and stir in the spirulina powder, sesame oil, salt, and chia seeds. Keep covered and allow to cool while you prepare the mushrooms.

2. To prepare the enoki, combine all enoki ingredients in a small bowl, tossing to coat well. Place a medium skillet over medium-high heat. Add the mushrooms and cook for 2 minutes, carefully turning them with tongs a couple of times.

3. Spread a sheet of nori on top of a sushi mat. Carefully spread ¼ cup quinoa on top, leaving about 2 inches uncovered at one end of the nori. An inch from the end closest to you, start adding your toppings

on top of the quinoa: one-quarter of the mushrooms, cucumbers, and avocado, and 1 scallion. Roll tightly, then seal the end by moistening the exposed part of the nori with water using your hands.

4. Repeat with the remaining rolls. Slice thin, using a sharp knife. Serve immediately.

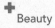
Beauty

Creamy Morel and Onion Dip

French onion dip gets an upgrade with dried morels. The trick to quickly browning the onions is to start with sugar. It adds a depth that's irresistible when combined with the slightly smoky dried morels. Dairy can cause congestion for some people, so this dip can be completely dairy-free if desired. If you'd prefer to omit the mayonnaise, replace it with 1 tablespoon more lemon juice.

SERVES: 6 to 8 | PREP AND COOK TIME: 30 minutes

½ ounce dried morel mushrooms, broken into small pieces and soaked in boiling water for 15 minutes

1 tablespoon sugar

3 large yellow onions, finely chopped

2 medium shallots, minced

¾ cup water, divided

1 tablespoon safflower oil

1 teaspoon salt

½ cup Greek yogurt, or silken tofu pureed with 1 tablespoon lemon juice

2 tablespoons mayonnaise

2 tablespoons nutritional yeast or grated Parmesan cheese

1 tablespoon lemon juice

1 teaspoon Worcestershire sauce

¼ cup minced flat-leaf parsley, or snipped chives

crackers or crudités, for serving

1. Drain the morels, straining and reserving the soaking water. Set aside.

2. Place the sugar, onions, and shallot in a medium stock pot over medium-high heat. Stir to combine and cook for 5 minutes, stirring occasionally. Add ¼ cup of the water and stir to deglaze the pan. Add the oil and salt, and cook another 5 minutes, adding more water if the mixture seems like it's getting too dark. Add ½ cup of the reserved soaking water, remaining ½ cup fresh water, and the morels.

3. Cover and let cook for another 5 minutes, being mindful that you have good ventilation and are not leaning over the pot. There should be little water left. If you have more than 2 tablespoons or so of liquid, continue cooking until it has evaporated. Remove the stockpot from the heat and let cool slightly.

4. Combine the remaining ingredients in a medium bowl, then add the slightly cooled onion mixture. Cover and refrigerate until completely cool.

5. Before serving, fold in the parsley or chives. Serve with crackers or crudités. This dip is especially good with bitter endive leaves.

✚ Immune

Garlicky Cremini-Shiitake Artichoke Dip

I love spinach and artichoke dip, but it can be heavy and its flavor flat, with no contrast, just rich creaminess. This double mushroom-artichoke version is just as creamy (yet dairy-free!), with much more flavor. Artichokes are high in antioxidants and are a traditional liver-supporting food. That's why I paired them with shiitakes here, plus a cashew cream in place of cheese and milk. It's also excellent tossed with hot pasta and some reserved cooking water for a pasta sauce.

SERVES: 4 to 6 | PREP AND COOK TIME: 20 minutes

1 cup raw cashews, soaked in hot water for at least 15 minutes

¾ cup mushroom broth

2 tablespoons lemon juice

1 tablespoon safflower oil

6 cloves garlic, minced

¼ teaspoon black pepper

1 teaspoon dried basil or oregano

1 cup sliced cremini mushrooms

4 shiitake mushroom caps, thinly sliced

16 ounces frozen artichoke hearts, thawed and finely chopped

1 teaspoon arrowroot powder

¼ cup nutritional yeast

½ teaspoon salt

chopped parsley, for garnish

baguette slices, pasta, or crudités, for serving

1. Drain the cashews, add to a blender, and blend until finely chopped.

2. Add the mushroom broth and lemon juice to the blender, and blend until completely smooth, pausing to scrape down the sides as needed. Set aside.

3. Place a medium saucepan over medium heat and add the safflower oil when the pan is hot. Add the garlic and cook for 2 minutes, stirring often.

4. Add the pepper, basil or oregano, and cremini and shiitakes. Cover and the raise heat to medium-high. Cook for about 5 minutes, stirring occasionally, until the mushrooms are tender.

5. Reduce the heat to medium-low, then stir in the cashew mixture, artichokes, arrowroot, and nutritional yeast. Cook, stirring often, until the mixture is bubbling and thickens slightly, about 3 minutes.

6. Remove from the heat, and season with salt to taste. Sprinkle with the chopped parsley and serve with baguette slices, over pasta, or with crudités for dipping.

✚
Detox, Immune

Basic Mushroom Duxelles

Infuse flavor into any dish with duxelles, a classic French recipe base. It's a mixture of finely chopped mushrooms, alliums, and herbs sauteed in butter or oil. You can change it up based on the mushrooms, alcohol, and fats you have on hand. Use a tablespoon or two in any dish that would benefit from a rich, savory flavor boost. Freeze leftovers in ice cube trays, then transfer to a sealed storage bag.

SERVES: 4 to 6 | PREP AND COOK TIME: 30 minutes

¼ cup safflower oil, divided

1 pound tender mushrooms, caps only, finely chopped

¼ cup minced shallots or 2 tablespoons minced garlic or ½ cup finely diced yellow onion

½ cup dry red or white wine, or ¼ cup dry sherry, divided

salt and pepper, to taste

1. Place a large saucepan over medium-high heat, then add 2 tablespoons of the safflower oil. Once hot, add the mushrooms and shallots, garlic, or onions and a pinch each of salt and pepper. Cook for 5 minutes, stirring often, until the mixture is dry and starting to get some color.

2. Add about half of the wine or sherry, stirring and scraping to remove any brown bits from the bottom of the pan.

3. Once the liquid has evaporated, add the remaining 2 tablespoons oil and another generous pinch each of salt and pepper. Continue cooking, stirring often, for another 5 minutes. If the shallots are in danger of burning, lower the heat to medium. Add the remaining wine or sherry, scraping the bottom as before, and cook until completely evaporated.

4. Let cool, then season to taste with salt and pepper. Refrigerate for up to 5 days or freeze for up to 3 months.

✚
Immune

Stuffed Maitake

Maitake are juicy and rich, which is why I love stuffing them with savory breadcrumbs. The crisp golden crust provides a wonderful contrast to the tender mushrooms. Don't be afraid to slice into the base of the maitake to make more room for the filling. It will hold together just fine as it bakes. Use this technique for lion's mane fillets, portobello caps, or oyster clusters.

SERVES: 4 | PREP AND COOK TIME: 45 minutes

2 (3.5-ounce) packages maitake mushrooms

1 cup fresh breadcrumbs

¼ cup grated Parmesan cheese, or 2 tablespoons nutritional yeast and 2 tablespoons ground cashews

2 tablespoons olive oil

2 cloves garlic, minced

½ teaspoon salt, divided

¼ teaspoon black pepper, divided

1 cup dry white wine

minced parsley, for garnish

1. Preheat the oven to 375°F.

2. Grease a baking dish with a neutral-flavored oil. Place the maitake in the prepared dish, and carefully open the petals. Use a paring knife to slice into the bases, leaving about ¼ inch at the bottom uncut. If the mushrooms fall into pieces, that's fine; just nestle them close together. Season with half the salt and pepper.

3. In a medium bowl, combine the breadcrumbs, Parmesan or nutritional yeast and cashews, olive oil, garlic, and remaining salt and pepper. The mixture will slightly stick together. Pack the breadcrumbs into and on top of the mushrooms. Pour the wine into the dish.

4. Bake for 30 to 35 minutes, until the crumb topping is golden brown and the mushrooms are cooked through. Garnish with parsley and serve immediately.

✚ Blood Sugar, Immune

Mixed Mushroom Pâté

This pâté concentrates the flavor of mushrooms, turning them into a rich sandwich spread or appetizer. In lieu of cream or butter, I swapped in creamy, buttery white beans for extra fiber and protein. This pâté is delicious paired with cucumber slices, the Gluten-Free Herbed Mushroom crackers on page 166, or thin slices of sourdough.

SERVES: 4 to 6 | PREP AND COOK TIME: 20 minutes

1 tablespoon safflower oil

¼ cup (½ stick) butter or safflower oil, divided

2 pounds mushrooms, such as button, cremini, shiitake, maitake, and/or oyster, finely chopped

3 shallots, minced

1 teaspoon dried tarragon

1 teaspoon dried chervil

¼ cup dry sherry, divided

1 cup mushroom broth

1 (14.5-ounce) can white beans, drained and rinsed

¼ cup flat-leaf parsley, minced

salt and pepper, to taste

1. Warm the safflower oil in a large saucepan over medium-high heat. Once hot, add half the butter or oil, the mushrooms, shallots, tarragon, chervil, and a pinch each of salt and pepper. Cook for 5 minutes, stirring often, until the mixture is dry and starting to get some color.

2. Add about half of the sherry, stirring and scraping to remove any brown bits from the bottom of the pan. Once the liquid has evaporated, add the remaining butter or oil and another generous pinch each of salt and pepper. Continue cooking, stirring often, for another 5 minutes. If the shallots are in danger of burning, lower heat to medium.

3. Add the remaining sherry, scraping the bottom as before, and cook until completely evaporated. Then add the broth and continue to cook over medium-high heat until mixture has reduced by half, about 2 minutes. Remove from the heat and let cool slightly.

4. Place the white beans in a food processor and process until completely smooth. Add the mushroom mixture and continue processing until all is completely smooth, then season to taste with salt and pepper. Add the parsley and pulse just to combine.

5. Line a loaf pan with parchment, and pour in the pâté, smoothing the top and pressing down firmly.

6. Cover and refrigerate for at least a few hours before serving so it firms up slightly. The pâté can be refrigerated up to 5 days or frozen for up to 3 months.

Immune

Spicy Maitake and Veggie-Stuffed Avocados

Calling all avocado lovers: Crunchy veggies and tender, spicy mushrooms are delightful on their own and even better when stuffed into and heaped onto half an avocado. This meal is low-carb too, which is why I used maitake—to help support healthy blood sugar levels.

SERVES: 4 | PREP AND COOK TIME: 25 minutes

2 teaspoons safflower oil

1 (3.5-ounce) package maitake mushrooms, chopped

1 tablespoon salt-free taco seasoning

¼ cup chopped red onion

¼ cup water

3 cloves garlic, minced

1 medium red or yellow bell pepper, diced

½ cup corn kernels

2 avocados, halved and pitted

¼ cup chopped cilantro leaves

2 tablespoons pumpkin seeds

1 lime, cut into wedges

salt and pepper, to taste

1. Place a medium skillet over medium-high heat. Add the safflower oil, along with the maitake, taco seasoning, and red onion. Cook, stirring occasionally, for about 5 minutes, until the onions start to get some color and soften. Add the water and cook another 5 minutes, until the water has mostly evaporated. Add the garlic, bell pepper, and corn, then lower the heat to medium. Cook another 5 minutes, until mixture is slightly softened and starting to get some color. Season to taste with salt and pepper.

2. To serve, scoop each avocado half out of the skin and place pit-side up on a plate. Top with a quarter of the maitake mixture. Garnish with the cilantro, pumpkin seeds, and lime wedges.

✚ Blood Sugar, Immune

Burdock-Shiitake Salad

This salad combines shiitake with burdock root, which is traditionally used to support the liver, plus cucumber and avocado for a side that's great for the skin. The dish needs no dressing; it starts with a traditional sweet and salty braise commonly used in Korean cooking. Serve over brown rice if desired. Burdock root is available at Asian markets and in most larger supermarkets. It will immediately begin to discolor when you peel it, and that's OK. It will not impact the flavor.

SERVES: 4 to 6 | PREP AND COOK TIME: 30 minutes

1 or 2 burdock roots (about 4 ounces each)

1 teaspoon regular sesame oil

4 shiitake mushroom caps, thinly sliced

2 tablespoons toasted sesame oil

2 tablespoons tamari

1 tablespoon sugar or honey

¼ teaspoon crushed red pepper or ½ teaspoon gochugaru (Korean chili powder)

¼ cup water

1 English cucumber, thinly sliced

1 avocado, pitted and diced

2 scallions, white and green parts, thinly sliced

2 tablespoons toasted sesame seeds

1. Prepare the burdock. Use a vegetable peeler to remove the dark outer skin, then julienne or shred the root using a food processor.

2. Place a medium skillet over medium-high heat. Add the regular sesame oil, then add the burdock and shiitakes. Cook, stirring often, for about 4 minutes, until the burdock starts to get some color.

3. Add the toasted sesame oil, tamari, sugar, and crushed red pepper or gochugaru, along with the water. Reduce the heat to medium, cover, and let simmer for 10 minutes, until the sauce has reduced and the burdock is tender but still chewy.

4. Remove from heat, and allow to cool for 10 minutes.

5. Toss the burdock and shiitakes, along with any sauce, with the remaining ingredients and serve immediately.

✚ Beauty, Detox, Immune

Shiitake and Edamame with Tahini Sauce

Shiitake and edamame pair well together, and their unique nutrition profiles also work synergistically. As it turns out, simmering (decocting) shiitakes in water or broth for six to eight minutes releases thioproline, also known as TCA, a natural antioxidant found in the liver. TCA helps neutralize the cancer-causing potential of nitrates and nitrites (found in processed meats like bacon and salami)—and protects against damage from acetaminophen. When foods containing TCA, like shiitakes, are cooked with foods containing cysteine, like both edamame and sesame, it helps increase TCA.[57] Of course, feel free to ignore the science behind it and just pair shiitakes and edamame because they taste delicious together! Healthy eating doesn't have to be complicated.

SERVES: 4 | PREP AND COOK TIME: 30 minutes

1 tablespoon safflower oil

1 cup thinly sliced shiitake mushrooms, caps only

¼ cup dry sherry

1 cup mushroom broth

1 tablespoon tamari

4 cloves garlic, minced

1 teaspoon cornstarch (optional)

½ cup water

2 tablespoons tahini

2 cups shelled frozen edamame, thawed

salt and pepper, to taste

toasted sesame seeds, for garnish

1. Heat a large skillet over medium-high heat. Add the oil, then add the shiitakes. Cook, stirring often, for 5 minutes, until the mushrooms start to darken and smell fragrant and earthy. Add the sherry, and scrape the bottom of the pan to release any brown bits from the pan. Add the mushroom broth, tamari, and garlic, reduce the heat to medium-low, then cover and let cook for 10 minutes.

2. After 10 minutes, whisk the cornstarch, if using, with the water and tahini. Whisk into the mushroom mixture, then add the edamame. Cook, stirring often, for about 2 minutes, until the edamame are heated through. Season to taste with salt and pepper.

3. Serve immediately, garnished with toasted sesame seeds.

✚ Beauty, Cholesterol, Detox, Immune

Look at the Big Picture

Don't get caught up in the details. When it comes to nutrition, look at the big picture, not the fine print. Reductionist nutrition is a popular approach to healthy eating, one that singles out foods for a single nutrient or attribute. You've likely seen this happen with foods like turmeric—we prize those curcumins for reducing inflammation! As a writer and health coach, there's a fine line for me between offering facts on a food's nutrient profile and painting it as *the* source of a certain nutrient or the fountain of youth. That even applies to mushrooms.

When I get caught up in the hype of whatever nutrient is trendy today, I take a deep breath and a step back, focusing on eating a varied, plant-based diet. Mushrooms are spectacular, but nothing should replace a healthy diet based on whole foods, plenty of moderate exercise, sufficient restful sleep, and healthy stress management.

Mushroom Cabbage Wraps

Swapping in cabbage leaves for rice or starchy wraps not only boosts your veggie intake for the day, it also keeps this dish lower in carbs. A 2015 study in the journal **Nutrients** *associated staple Nordic foods like cabbage with a reduced risk of type-2 diabetes.[58] I don't have a problem with carbs, but I do love cabbage and all its cruciferous brethren, and I think wrapping food in crunchy cabbage leaves is a fun way to eat!*

SERVES: 4 | PREP AND COOK TIME: 30 minutes

1 tablespoon regular sesame oil

4 ounces minced shiitake mushrooms

4 ounces white button or bunapi mushrooms

8 ounces firm tofu, mashed

4 cloves garlic, minced

2 teaspoons grated fresh ginger

1 carrot, peeled and julienned

½ cup prepared kimchi, drained and finely chopped

1 tablespoon hoisin sauce

1 teaspoon tamari

¼ teaspoon crushed red pepper (optional)

4 scallions, white and green parts, minced, divided

1 teaspoon toasted sesame oil

12 Napa cabbage leaves

2 tablespoons toasted sesame seeds, for garnish

1. Place a skillet over medium-high heat. Add the oil, then add the shiitakes, white buttons or bunapis, and tofu. Cook, stirring often, for about 5 minutes, until the mushrooms and tofu start to get some color. Add the remaining ingredients, reserving 2 tablespoons of the scallions, the cabbage leaves, and the sesame seeds, and lower the heat to medium. Cook, stirring often, for up to 10 minutes, until most of the moisture has evaporated.

2. While the mushroom mixture is cooking, steam the Napa cabbage leaves in a pot with a little boiling water for 30 seconds (for crisper cabbage) to 1 minute (for more tender cabbage), then shock in an ice water bath. Drain well.

3. Once the mushroom mixture is cooked, arrange the cabbage leaves on a platter. Divide the mushroom mixture among the cabbage leaves, then top with the remaining scallions and the sesame seeds.

✚ Detox, Immune

Seared Maitake

This dish was inspired by one from one of my favorite restaurants, Plant in Asheville. It's a simple preparation that highlights the savory yet light flavor of maitake. The trick is get your pan nice and hot, then press those mushrooms so the edges get brown and crispy.

SERVES: 4 | PREP AND COOK TIME: 10 minutes

2 tablespoons safflower oil

2 (3.5-ounce) packages maitake mushrooms, halved

½ cup dry white wine or ¼ cup dry sherry

2 cloves garlic, minced

salt and pepper, to taste

1. Place a medium skillet over medium-high heat. Once hot, add the oil.

2. Season the maitake liberally with salt and pepper. Place them in the skillet, cut side down.

3. Cook for 3 minutes, occasionally pressing down firmly with a metal spatula. Carefully turn them, then cook another 3 minutes.

4. Add the wine or sherry and garlic, then scrape the bottom of the pan to remove any brown bits from the pan. Lower the heat to medium and cook for about 2 minutes more to allow the sauce to reduce slightly. Remove from heat and serve immediately.

✚
Blood Sugar, Immune

Oyster Mushroom Orzo

This humble orzo dish is right at home alongside roasted root vegetables in the fall and winter months. With fragrant sage and plenty of oyster and shiitake mushrooms, each bite of al dente orzo is bursting with flavor. You can swap in quinoa (try red, as it stays firmer) or pearled barley if desired.

SERVES: 4 | PREP AND COOK TIME: 20 minutes

1 tablespoon safflower oil

1 medium yellow onion, finely chopped

1 teaspoon sage, thinly sliced

¼ teaspoon black pepper

½ pound oyster mushrooms, roughly chopped

1 shiitake mushroom cap, thinly sliced

1 ounce dry sherry

1½ cups whole wheat orzo

3 cups mushroom broth

2 tablespoons nutritional yeast or grated Parmesan cheese

1. Place a medium saucepan over medium-high heat. Warm the oil, then add the onions. Sauté, stirring often, for about 5 minutes, until the onions have softened slightly and started to brown. Add the sage, pepper, and mushrooms, and sauté another 5 minutes, stirring occasionally.

2. Pour in the sherry to deglaze the pan, scraping the bottom to loosen any brown bits. Stir in the orzo, then add the broth. Increase the heat to high, bring to a boil, then reduce the heat to low. Cover and allow to simmer for 10 minutes.

3. Remove from the heat, stir in the nutritional yeast or Parmesan cheese, and let sit for 5 minutes. Fluff with a fork and serve immediately.

✚ Cholesterol, Beauty, Mood

Mushroom "Escargots"

The best part about the classic French entree escargots is the irresistible garlic-parsley butter sauce. Mushrooms easily stand in for snails, and the sauce turns even simple button mushrooms into a decadent start to a meal. This recipe felt right, since both snails and mushrooms are found on the forest floor. You can also swap in shiitake caps or maitake petals.

SERVES: 4 | PREP AND COOK TIME: 30 minutes

1 tablespoon safflower oil

¼ cup (½ stick) butter or olive oil

8 cloves garlic, minced

1 medium shallot, minced

1 pound cremini or white button mushrooms, stems discarded

¼ teaspoon salt, plus more to taste

¼ teaspoon black pepper, plus more to taste

pinch of ground nutmeg

½ cup dry white wine

½ cup flat-leaf parsley, finely chopped

zest and juice of ½ lemon

toasted baguette slices, for serving

1. Place a medium skillet over medium heat. Add the oil and butter, if using, then, once hot and melted, add the garlic and shallot. Cook, stirring often, for about 5 minutes, until they are soft and starting to get some color. Add the mushrooms, salt, pepper, and nutmeg. Cover and cook for 10 minutes, stirring and flipping the mushrooms occasionally.

2. Increase the heat to medium-high, add the wine, and scrape the bottom of the pan to remove any brown bits. Remove from the heat and add the parsley. Season to taste with more salt, pepper, and the lemon zest and juice. Serve immediately, with baguette slices for dipping.

✚
Immune

Mushroom Pilaf

Mushrooms give this toasted rice dish a boost. To give it more contrast and nutrition, I've added currants and walnuts. You could also serve it over a bed of arugula or with a poached egg or seared tofu for a full meal. This dish is in regular rotation at my house, and I often swap in different types of dried fruit, nuts, and fresh herbs depending on what I have on hand.

SERVES: 4 to 6 | PREP AND COOK TIME: 1 hour

1 tablespoon safflower oil

1 medium yellow onion, diced

½ teaspoon dried thyme

1 (8-ounce) package tender mushrooms, sliced

2 cups medium-grain brown rice

½ cup dry white wine

1 teaspoon tamari

2½ cups mushroom or vegetable broth

2 tablespoons orange juice

1 tablespoon orange zest

¼ cup dried currants

½ cup chopped walnuts

¼ cup chopped flat-leaf parsley

1. Place a large saucepan over medium-high heat, then add the oil. Add the onion, thyme, and mushrooms. Cook, stirring occasionally, for about 5 minutes, until the onions and mushrooms start to darken.

2. Stir in the rice and cook for 1 minute, until fragrant and toasty. Add the wine, stir to combine, and scrape up any brown bits from the bottom of the pan.

3. Add the tamari and broth, increase the heat to high, and bring to a boil. Immediately reduce the heat to low, cover, and cook for 35 to 40 minutes, until rice is tender.

4. Remove from heat, fluff with a fork, and mix in the remaining ingredients, then serve immediately.

+ Immune

Shiitake Sauerkraut

I took a workshop with legendary fermenter Sandor Katz a couple of years ago, and he opened my eyes to fermenting beyond basic kimchi and sauerkraut. With Katz's guidance in mind, I started fermenting shiitakes in my veggie blends last year. I enjoy a spoonful every morning with breakfast, usually on top of avocado toast. Note that even here we aren't eating the mushrooms raw—we're boiling them, letting them cool, then fermenting with the cabbage. Tip: Don't discard the juice. Take shots of it daily or mix into salad dressings.

SERVES: 4 to 6 | PREP AND COOK TIME: 30 minutes, plus 7 to 10 days to ferment

1 cup fresh shiitake caps, sliced, or dried shiitakes, broken into small pieces

1 to 3 tablespoons salt, divided

1 small head purple cabbage, shredded

1 teaspoon caraway or cumin seeds (optional)

1. Place the shiitakes in a medium saucepan and cover with filtered water by 1 inch.

2. Bring to a boil and cook for 10 minutes. Stir in 1 tablespoon of the salt. Let cool completely.

3. Place the cabbage in a large, deep bowl, then pour the liquid from the shiitakes on top. Massage and squeeze the cabbage until it starts to release its juices. Taste for salt and add more if desired.

4. Mix in the shiitakes and caraway or cumin seeds, if using, and transfer the mixture to a quart-size jar. Press the cabbage and shiitakes down firmly so they all fit in the jar and are submerged. Use a small glass jar on top to keep everything submerged. Weigh down the top of the sauerkraut, and cover with a cloth or fermentation lid.

5. Allow to ferment at room temperature for 7 to 10 days, until the sauerkraut is bubbling and tangy. Refrigerate for up to 3 months.

Detox, Cholesterol, Skin

Korean-Style Marinated Shiitake Mushrooms

The best part of any Korean meal, in my opinion, is **banchan**, the side dishes. You get to sample several different foods, which is wonderful way to diversify any healthy diet. Marinated shiitakes are a common Korean side. This is a good recipe for dried shiitakes, which have a meaty, hearty texture after being reconstituted. You can adjust the marinade as desired, adding more or fewer salty, sweet, or acidic ingredients to suit your palate.

SERVES: 4 to 6 | PREP AND COOK TIME: 30 minutes

1 quart (4 cups) water

8 to 12 dried shiitake mushrooms

½ teaspoon sea salt or tamari

1 tablespoon gochugaru (Korean chili powder)

1 tablespoon rice vinegar

1 garlic clove, minced

1 tablespoon maple syrup or brown sugar

1 tablespoon toasted sesame oil

1 teaspoon toasted sesame seeds

1. Bring the water to a boil in large saucepan. Add the mushrooms and salt or tamari, and simmer until tender, about 10 minutes. Drain, reserving the cooking water.

2. Allow the mushrooms to cool slightly, then thinly slice.

3. Combine the red pepper, vinegar, garlic, maple syrup or brown sugar, sesame oil, and sesame seeds in a shallow dish. Add the mushrooms and toss to combine. Add a couple of tablespoons of the cooking water, reserving the rest for another purpose if desired.

4. Cover, marinate, and refrigerate for 15 minutes or up to overnight. These taste better the longer they sit in the marinade.

✚ Detox, Cholesterol, Skin

Tender Mushroom Gravy

This mushroom gravy is a family favorite, and it goes quickly at holiday gatherings. Serve it alongside lean cuts of meat or vegetarian dishes for a drizzle of flavor and umami. Sautéing the mushrooms until they're nice and brown, then adding rich tamari and tangy nutritional yeast are the secrets to this delectable gravy. Bonus: Since it contains no meat, it's cholesterol-free!

SERVES: 4 to 6 | PREP AND COOK TIME: 30 minutes

2 tablespoons safflower oil

2 cups sliced tender mushrooms

1 medium yellow onion, diced

3 cloves garlic, minced

2 tablespoons dried rosemary, sage, or thyme, or any combination

2 tablespoons tamari

¼ cup (½ stick) butter or safflower oil

½ cup all-purpose flour or oat flour

¼ cup nutritional yeast

¼ teaspoon black pepper

1 cup mushroom broth

1. Place a large, deep skillet over medium-high heat. Add the oil, and once warm, add the mushrooms and onions. Cook, stirring often, for about 5 minutes, until the mixture starts to soften and get some color. Lower the heat to medium, then add the garlic and herbs. Cook another 2 minutes, then add the tamari and butter or oil. Once melted, add the flour, nutritional yeast and pepper. Cook, stirring often, for about 2 minutes more, until the mixture is toasty and fragrant.

2. Whisk in the broth. Simmer for 10 minutes, stirring constantly, until thick and creamy. Add water or more broth if you prefer a thinner gravy.

3. Serve immediately over biscuits, sautéed greens, or toast.

✚
Immune

CHAPTER 6

——————— ⊁ ———————

Main Dishes

As a longtime plant-based eater, I embrace mushrooms as a stand-alone main dish. At my dinner table, mushrooms can be the starring ingredient, both for flavor and nutrition. However, I know that not everyone feels that mushrooms are substantial enough to be at the center of the plate, so many of these recipes include other proteins too.

You'll find a balance of dishes in which mushrooms are the focus, as well as some where they're one of several key ingredients. And, while this chapter shares plenty of creative ways to introduce unique or seasonal tender mushrooms to your plate, it also contains comforting recipes featuring common mushrooms.

Slow Cooker Medicinal Mushroom Soup

Slow-cooked soups are one of my favorite ways to enjoy mushrooms, and in the winter months, I keep my immune system fortified by including medicinal herbs too. Here, I used red ginseng, which helps keep your body from being overstimulated, and astragalus, a Chinese root that's my go-to for building up my immune system and keeping it strong throughout cold and flu season. I also included jujubes, or red dates, which are often used as a tonic in TCM (similar to ginseng). I switch up the tough mushroom (reishi, cordyceps, or turkey tail) I use based on what I have on hand, and you can use more than one if you have them.

SERVES: 4 | PREP AND COOK TIME: 8½ hours

1 tablespoon safflower oil

1 large yellow onion, diced

1 pound tender mushrooms, sliced

4 cloves garlic, minced

1-inch piece red ginseng

2 pieces astragalus

4 jujubes

1 slice reishi, 1 teaspoon ground cordyceps (or 1 or 2 dried), and/ or 1 turkey tail

1 teaspoon salt, plus more to taste

1 cup brown rice

¼ cup white miso paste

1 pound firm tofu or 1 (5-ounce) package fresh yuba, diced, for serving

thinly sliced scallions, for serving

black pepper, to taste

1. Set a slow cooker or multicooker to sauté. (Or saute in a pan on the stove.) Add the oil, then add the onions and tender mushrooms. Cook, stirring occasionally, until the onions soften, about 5 minutes. Add the garlic, ginseng, astragalus, jujubes, reishi, cordyceps and/or turkey tail, 1 teaspoon salt, and rice. Cover with water to the max-fill line of your pot.

2. Set on low heat for 8 hours.

3. Before serving, whisk in the miso, season to taste with salt and pepper, and stir in the tofu and scallions.

✚ Adaptogenic, Energy, Immune, Sleep, Stress

Chinese Chicken Soup with Herbs and Cordyceps

I firmly believe in the power of eating more plants (and mushrooms, of course), and this recipe from Abby Artemisia illustrates how you can integrate more wild plants and mushrooms into a standard American diet. She uses a single chicken breast for an entire pot of soup, which supports both her own philosophy on animal products as well as that of TCM. That is, use small amounts of high-quality animal protein medicinally. Abby paired cordyceps with herbs that tonify the qi (chi). They help rebuild vital energy, and correct imbalances and deficiencies. Visit your local herb store or co-op to find the herbs she used. Note: Since it is challenging to find whole dried cordyceps, Abby opted to use powdered dried mushrooms instead. This is not the same as powdered cordyceps extract, which has already been processed and doesn't need the lengthy cooking time.

SERVES: 4 | PREP AND COOK TIME: 1 hour, plus overnight for soaking

10 dried jujubes

¼ cup dried wild yam pieces

¼ cup dried goji berries

1 tablespoon powdered cordyceps mushrooms (see note)

1 cup fresh lotus root slices

1 cup bamboo shoots

2½ quarts (10 cups) chicken bone broth

1 medium chicken breast (on the bone will give more flavor, but boneless is fine)

salt, to taste (optional)

1. In a large stock pot, soak all the ingredients except for the chicken in the broth overnight in the refrigerator.

2. Add the chicken and simmer for 1 hour. Remove the chicken, shred or dice it, then return the meat to the pot. Season with salt to taste, if desired.

✚ Adaptogenic, Energy, Immune, Stress

Potato, Leek, and Oyster Mushroom Soup

In this classic soup, oyster mushrooms are cooked a long while to allow their flavor to intensify, adding a bit more depth to this smooth, simple soup. Oyster mushrooms are traditionally used to lower cholesterol, so I opted to omit the traditional heavy cream, instead blending cashews with some of the soup. Without the cashews, the soup is still tasty but isn't quite as creamy.

SERVES: 6 | PREP AND COOK TIME: 1 hour

1 tablespoon safflower oil

2 leeks, white and light green parts only, thinly sliced

2 cups oyster mushrooms, chopped

½ cup dry white wine

1 tablespoon fresh tarragon, finely chopped

1 teaspoon salt

¼ teaspoon black pepper

3 medium Yukon gold potatoes, diced (peeling is optional)

1 bay leaf

1 quart (4 cups) mushroom broth

1 quart (4 cups) water

¼ cup raw cashews soaked in hot water for at least 15 minutes (optional)

1 tablespoon lemon juice

snipped chives, for garnish

1. Place a large stock pot over medium-high heat. Add the oil, and once hot, add the leeks and oyster mushrooms. Cook, stirring often, for about 10 minutes, until they are softened and getting plenty of color. (If the mixture starts to get too dark too soon, add a splash of mushroom broth or water and scrape the bottom of the pan.)

2. Add the wine, scraping the bottom of the pan to release any brown bits, then stir in the tarragon. Add the salt, pepper, and potatoes, stir to combine, then add the bay leaf, mushroom broth, and water. Bring to a boil, then cover, reduce the heat to medium-low, and simmer for 30 minutes. Then remove from the heat.

3. Drain the cashews, if using. Transfer the cashews and the lemon juice along with 2 cups of the soup to a blender. Process until completely smooth. Pour the pureed soup back into the pot and stir to combine.

4. Serve immediately, garnished with snipped chives, if desired. Refrigerate for up to 3 days or freeze up to 3 months.

✚ Cholesterol, Mood, Skin

Tofu, Hijiki, and Shiitake Stir-Fry

Creamy tofu, earthy shiitakes, and briny hijiki are a study in contrast in this quick stir-fry. Seaweeds—or sea vegetables, as I prefer to call them—are wonderful sources of essential minerals, and they add an oceanlike flavor to dishes. Hijiki, a brown seaweed that grows on rocky coastlines in Korea and Japan, is traditionally used to support the thyroid and healthy blood sugar levels. In Japan, hijiki is prized as a food to increase beauty. If you can't find it, use an equal amount of arame or wakame.

SERVES: 4 | PREP AND COOK TIME: 30 minutes

2 tablespoons safflower oil

1 pound firm tofu, cubed and pressed to remove excess water

1 cup sliced shiitake caps

1 bunch scallions, thinly sliced, white and green parts separated

1 ounce dry sherry or mushroom broth

3 medium carrots, peeled and sliced into ½-inch rounds

1 pound fresh broccoli, stems trimmed and broken into florets

½ cup water, divided

½ cup hijiki, soaked in cool water for 30 minutes, drained and rinsed

black sesame seeds, for garnish

For the sauce:

1½ teaspoons toasted sesame oil

1 tablespoon black bean and garlic paste

1 teaspoon grated fresh ginger

1 teaspoon tamari

1 tablespoon maple syrup

¼ teaspoon crushed red pepper

½ teaspoon arrowroot powder

1. Place a large wok or deep skillet over medium-high heat, then add the oil. Add the tofu and cook until golden brown on all sides, about 10 minutes. (Turn the tofu when it's easy to move; if it's still stuck to the pan, it's not ready.) Remove from the pan and set aside.

2. Add the shiitakes and the white parts of the scallions. Cook for about 3 minutes, until the mushrooms darken and the onions get some color. Add the sherry and immediately scrape the bottom of the pan to remove any brown bits. Add the carrots, broccoli, and ¼ cup of the water. Cover and let cook about 5 minutes, until the vegetables are

tender but crisp. Meanwhile, combine all ingredients for the sauce in a small bowl.

3. Lower the heat to medium, then stir in the hijiki and the sauce. Add the tofu back to the dish with the remaining ¼ cup water. Cook for about 5 minutes, until the sauce is bubbling and slightly thickened.

4. Remove from the heat and serve immediately, garnished with the sesame seeds and green parts of the scallions.

✚
Beauty, Cholesterol, Detox, Skin

Lion's Mane Fillets

This is a method more than a recipe; it's how I usually start out cooking lion's mane. Once you get a nice brown crust on the outside, you can use them in any dish, just as you would chicken breasts or mild white fish fillets. Don't let lion's mane's shaggy appearance deter you from buying and preparing it. I was nervous that I'd mess up this glorious mushroom, but it's quite simple to cook—and the results are so worth it!

SERVES: 4 | PREP AND COOK TIME: 20 minutes

1 pound lion's mane mushrooms, sliced into ¾-inch fillets, excess water pressed out

1 tablespoon safflower oil

½ cup dry white wine or 2 tablespoons dry sherry

1 medium shallot or 3 cloves garlic, minced

salt and pepper, to taste

1. Season the lion's mane with salt and pepper.

2. Place a large skillet over medium-high heat. Add the oil, then place the lion's mane fillets in the skillet in a single layer with at least one inch between each one. Cook them in batches if necessary.

3. Use a metal spatula to press down firmly on the lion's mane as it cooks. After 3 minutes, it should be nicely browned. If it's not, continue cooking until it is as dark as you'd like it to be. Flip and cook another 3 minutes, continuing to press down firmly.

4. Lower the heat to medium, then add the wine or sherry and shallot or garlic. Cover and cook for about 2 minutes, until the shallots or garlic have softened and the wine or sherry have reduced. Season with salt and pepper to taste and serve immediately.

VARIATIONS

- Season with ⅛ teaspoon kelp granules for "fish" fillets.

- Add ¼ cup pitted kalamata olives, 2 tablespoons chopped sun-dried tomatoes, and 1 tablespoon lemon juice at the end.

- Add 1 tablespoon fresh dill or tarragon during the last 2 minutes of cooking.

- Stir in 2 tablespoons chimichurri or pesto.

- Swap for chicken in a piccata recipe.

- Let cool, then pull into strips and swap for tuna in any tuna salad recipe.

- Season with Italian herbs. Once seared, use in any chicken Parmesan recipe.

- Toss with barbecue sauce (though this does start to overpower the mushroom's lovely flavor).

- Dredge in seasoned batter and pan-fry it.

- Use it in place of the chicken in chicken and dumplings.

✚
Memory, Nervous System

Fajita Veggie-Stuffed Portobellos

Portobellos are hearty and meaty; they stand up well to heavy, intense spices and marinades, and are often included in fajitas. I decided to keep them whole and bake them with seared vegetables and a spicy tomato sauce. This is a recipe suitable for mushroom newbies or those who might be squeamish about some of the more exotic varieties.

SERVES: 4 | PREP AND COOK TIME: 1 hour, plus time to marinate

4 portobello caps

2 tablespoons salt-free taco seasoning

2 tablespoons apple cider vinegar

1 tablespoon safflower oil

¼ cup water

1 large green bell pepper, sliced into strips

1 medium red or yellow onion, sliced into strips

1 (14.5-ounce) can diced tomatoes

salt and pepper, to taste

1. Season the portobellos with salt and pepper on both sides. Place in an oven-proof baking dish, gill-sides up.

2. In a small bowl, mix the taco seasoning, vinegar, and oil together with the water, then pour evenly over the mushrooms. Marinate covered in the refrigerator for 1 hour or up to overnight.

3. Preheat the oven to 425°F.

4. Place a large skillet over high heat. Season the peppers and onions with salt and pepper.

5. Add the vegetables to the pan and cook for 1 minute without moving them around. Use tongs to toss and turn the vegetables and cook for another minute, until nicely darkened in some spots.

6. Remove from the heat and divide the vegetables into and around the mushrooms. Top each mushroom cap with 1 tablespoon of the diced tomatoes with juice, then pour the rest into the bottom of the dish.

7. Bake uncovered for 45 minutes, checking after 30 minutes to ensure all the liquid hasn't evaporated. If so, add ¼ cup water. When ready,

the mushrooms and vegetables will be tender, while the sauce will have thickened. Serve immediately.

+ Immune

Baked Salmon Fillets with Creamy Shiitake Sauce

Abby Artemisia never fails to surprise me with her unique use of foraged ingredients. Here, she uses evergreen needles to capture the essence and herbal flavor of the forest, plus wild onions and dried shiitakes. The dish is equally delicious with tofu or lion's mane fillets, and if you don't have evergreen needles on hand—I didn't when I made my tofu version—swap in an equal amount of rosemary.

SERVES: 4 | PREP AND COOK TIME: 30 minutes

2 tablespoons butter or olive oil, divided

4 (4-ounce) wild salmon fillets

1 cup dried shiitake mushrooms, quartered, soaked in hot water for at least 10 minutes

2 tablespoons coconut flour

1 tablespoon fresh or 1½ teaspoons dried fir, spruce, or pine needles, minced

2 tablespoons wild onions or scallions, minced or cut fine with kitchen scissors

1 teaspoon salt

½ cup milk

2 tablespoons lemon juice

1. Preheat the oven to 350°F. Drain the mushrooms and squeeze out as much water as possible.

2. Use 1 teaspoon of the butter or oil to grease a casserole dish large enough to hold all the salmon. Add the salmon fillets, skin-side down.

3. Place a medium skillet over medium heat. Add the butter or oil and, once melted, add the mushrooms. Cook for 1 minute, stirring often.

4. In a small bowl, combine the coconut flour, evergreen needles, onions, salt, and milk.

5. Add the milk mixture to the pan with the mushrooms and cook for 3 minutes, until warmed and starting to thicken. Whisk in the lemon juice and remove from the heat.

6. Spread the mushroom mixture evenly over the salmon. Bake for 15 to 25 minutes, until the fish is flaky. Serve immediately.

✚ Detox, Immune

White Bean, Mushroom, and Wild Rice Sauté

Creamy white beans add comfort to this easy meal. Other than the wild rice, this recipe contains ingredients that are already likely to be in your kitchen in the cooler months. This gluten-free grain is high in protein with a distinctly nutty taste and firm bite. Wild rice is native to North America and grows in shallow streams in the Great Lakes region.

SERVES: 4 | PREP AND COOK TIME: 1 hour

1 cup wild rice or wild rice blend

2 cups mushroom broth

1 bay leaf

1 tablespoon safflower oil

1 tablespoon butter

1 medium onion, diced

1 tablespoon fresh rosemary

1 teaspoon fresh thyme leaves

1 pint tender mushrooms, thinly sliced

3 medium carrots, peeled and sliced into ½-inch rounds

4 stalks celery, sliced into ½-inch pieces

1 (14.5-ounce) can white beans, drained and rinsed

1 tablespoon tamari

salt and pepper, to taste

1. Bring the rice, broth, and bay leaf to a boil in a medium saucepan.

2. Reduce the heat to a simmer, cover, and let simmer for 45 minutes, or until tender.

3. Meanwhile, place a large, deep skillet over medium heat. Add the oil and butter. Once melted, add the onion, rosemary, thyme, and pepper. Cook for about 5 minutes, until the onions start to soften.

4. Add the mushrooms, carrots, and celery. Cook for 6 to 8 minutes, until the carrots and celery are starting to get tender. Stir in the cooked rice, beans, and tamari. Cook another 3 minutes, until the beans are heated through. Season with salt and pepper to taste and serve immediately.

+ Immune

Oyster Mushroom Philly Cheesesteak Potatoes

These are definitely not traditional Philly cheesesteaks. First of all, there's no bun—just a baked potato. And there are oyster mushrooms in place of beef (your cholesterol levels thank you for that!). But I did keep all those tender-crisp onions and peppers, then finished it off with smoky Gouda (if you don't eat dairy or are watching your cholesterol, you can use the Follow Your Heart vegan version). This is another recipe for the mushroom skeptics out there.

SERVES: 4 | PREP AND COOK TIME: 1 hour

1 tablespoon red miso paste

1 tablespoon Worcestershire sauce

1 teaspoon maple syrup

¼ teaspoon black pepper

1 tablespoon apple cider vinegar

1 pound oyster mushrooms, pulled into bite-size pieces

1 tablespoon safflower oil

1 medium yellow onion, thinly sliced

2 medium bell peppers, any color, thinly sliced

3 cloves garlic, minced

4 ounces smoked Gouda

4 russet potatoes, baked or steamed

1. In a medium bowl, combine the miso, Worcestershire, maple syrup, pepper, and vinegar. Add the oyster mushrooms and toss to combine. Let marinate for 15 minutes.

2. Place a large cast-iron skillet over medium-high heat. Add the oil, then add the onion and peppers. Cook, stirring often, for about 3 minutes, until they start to get some color.

3. Lower the heat to medium, then add the mushrooms, reserving any marinade. Cook for 10 minutes, stirring often, until the mushrooms and vegetables are tender and getting some nice brown color.

4. Add the garlic and the marinade. Cook for about 2 minutes, until the garlic is softened and no longer raw. Add the cheese, then cover and cook until melted.

5. Split open the potatoes, fluffing the flesh with a fork. Divide the mushroom mixture over the tops of the potatoes. Serve immediately.

✚ Cholesterol, Mood, Skin

Slow Cooker Venison and Hen of the Woods Chili

Abby Artemisia is not only a successful herbalist and forager, she's also a mom, so she knows how family-friendly slow cooker dinners can be. She excitedly texted me about this recipe, as a way to introduce people to wild game. Her venison came from a local friend who hunts, but you can now find game at many co-ops and grocery stores. If you don't eat meat, swap in more beans or finely diced tender mushrooms.

SERVES: 6 to 8 | PREP AND COOK TIME: 8 hours, 15 minutes

1 cup dried maitake mushrooms, finely crumbled, soaked in 2 cups hot water for at least 10 minutes

1½ pounds venison roast or stew meat, cut into ½-inch cubes, or ground venison

½ pound ground beef or pork

1 (14.5-ounce) can kidney beans, drained and rinsed

1 large white onion, diced

1 or 2 jalapenos, or another hot pepper, diced

1 (14.5-ounce) can diced tomatoes

6 cloves garlic

2 tablespoons chili powder or salt-free taco seasoning

1 tablespoon fresh oregano or bee balm leaf

salt and pepper, to taste

1. Drain the mushrooms, reserving and straining the soaking water. Squeeze out as much water as possible from the mushrooms. Set aside.

2. Add all ingredients including the soaking water, except for salt and pepper, to a slow cooker.

3. Cover and cook on low for 8 hours.

4. Season to taste and serve immediately.

✚ Blood Sugar, Immune

Hen of the Woods Tacos

Combining mushrooms with ground meat is an easy way to introduce them to picky eaters. These easy, family-friendly tacos by Abby Artemisia are on the table in 30 minutes and make use of dried mushrooms. If you are lucky enough to find wild maitake (hen of the woods) mushrooms, preserve your harvest and use them in tacos all year round. If you, unlike Abby, are not a foraged foods expert, simply use fresh cultivated maitake.

SERVES: 4 | PREP AND COOK TIME: 30 minutes

1 cup dried maitake mushrooms, finely crumbled, soaked in hot water for at least 10 minutes and drained

1 tablespoon neutral oil

1 pound ground beef, ground turkey, or vegetarian crumbles

½ white onion, diced

1 to 2 tablespoons Mexican seasoning or chili powder

4 small cloves garlic, minced

8 taco shells

salt, to taste

For the toppings:

chopped green or wild onions

shredded cheese

sour cream

chopped lettuce

1. Drain the mushrooms and squeeze out as much water as possible.

2. Place a large skillet over medium low-heat, then add the oil. Once warm, add the ground beef, turkey, or vegetarian crumbles, and break into small crumbles as it cooks.

3. When the meat is about halfway done, add the mushrooms.

4. Cook, stirring frequently, for about 10 minutes total, until the meat starts to brown. Add the onions, Mexican seasoning or chili powder, and garlic, and cook until the meat is no longer pink. Remove from the heat and season to taste with salt.

5. Meanwhile, heat the taco shells in the oven according to the package directions.

6. Serve immediately with desired toppings.

✚ Blood Sugar, Immune

Lion's Mane Burgers

Abby Artemisia makes her living reconnecting people with nature, introducing them to the edible mushrooms and plants in their area. It used to be only by the grace of Mother Nature that either of us could enjoy lion's mane for supper. Now, thanks to growers like the Food Fight Farm in Mars Hill, North Carolina, this delicacy is more readily available. This is another dish that's great for new mushroom eaters.

You can actually use any mushroom in your burgers, up to a 50/50 mix. The umami in mushrooms allows you to reduce sodium, saturated fat, and cholesterol in ground meat dishes without impacting the flavor of a dish (and it helps you stay fuller longer).[59]

SERVES: 4 | PREP AND COOK TIME: 30 minutes

1 cup dried lion's mane mushrooms, soaked in 1 cup hot water for at least 15 minutes

1 tablespoon olive oil

4 cloves garlic, minced

1 teaspoon salt

1 pound ground beef

½ teaspoon black pepper

1. Drain the mushrooms and squeeze as much water from them as possible, then roughly chop.

2. Place a large skillet over medium heat. Add the mushrooms and cook for about 5 minutes, until heated through. Add the garlic and salt and cook for another for about 2 minutes more, until the garlic is fragrant and the mushrooms have released most of their water. Remove from the heat.

3. Place the ground beef in a large bowl, then fold in the mushrooms and season with the pepper. Use your hands to form 4 patties.

4. Place a grill pan or the same large skillet over medium-low heat. Once hot, cook the burgers for 10 minutes, or until they reach the desired level of doneness.

✚ Immune, Memory, Nervous System

Tempeh Steaks with Black Pepper–Mushroom Sauce

Black pepper is naturally heating, and it has traditionally been used to aid digestion. In this savory sauce, it perks up mushrooms and tempeh. Tempeh is a fermented soy protein that's native to Indonesia. The soybeans are inoculated with a fungus (so it's kind of like an honorary mushroom!), which makes the protein more digestible. I like Smiling Hara's Smoked Salt and Pepper Steak tempeh here, but if you're a meat eater, swap in your favorite protein.

SERVES: 4 | PREP AND COOK TIME: 30 minutes

2 tablespoons safflower oil

1 (8-ounce) block tempeh, quartered

2 cups sliced tender mushrooms

3 medium shallots, minced

1½ teaspoons black pepper, plus more to taste

¼ cup dry sherry

1 teaspoon tamari

2 tablespoons butter

2 tablespoons all-purpose or whole-wheat pastry flour

1 cup mushroom broth

¼ cup chopped flat-leaf parsley

salt, to taste

1. Place a medium skillet over medium-high heat. Add the oil, and once hot, add the tempeh. Cook for 2 minutes, then flip and cook another 1 to 2 minutes, until nicely browned and warmed through. Set aside.

2. Add the mushrooms, shallots, and black pepper to the pan. Cook, stirring often, for about 5 minutes, until they start to soften and get some color. Add the sherry, then scrape up any brown bits from the bottom of the pan.

3. Lower the heat to medium, add the butter and, once melted, add the flour. Stir constantly for about 2 minutes, until the flour is cooked and smells nutty. Add the stock, return the tempeh to the pan, cover, and cook for about 10 minutes, until the sauce has thickened nicely. Season with additional salt and pepper to taste.

4. Serve immediately, topped with parsley.

✚ Immune

Easy Mushroom Tostadas

I make these tostadas at least every week. They also satisfy my cravings for nachos—you could pile the ingredients on chips too. I like Frontier's Chili Powder Blend for the taco seasoning, but use whatever brand you like.

SERVES: 4 | PREP AND COOK TIME: 45 minutes

1 tablespoon safflower oil

1 (8-ounce package) tender mushrooms, sliced

1 large yellow onion, diced

1 red or yellow bell pepper, diced

3 cloves garlic, minced

1 tablespoon salt-free taco seasoning

1 tablespoon tomato paste

1 cup diced tomatoes

4 large tortillas, preferably whole-grain

4 cups baby kale or spinach

½ cup shredded cheese

1 avocado, diced

¼ cup chopped cilantro

sliced black olives and scallions, for garnish (optional)

salt, to taste

1. Place a large skillet over medium-high heat, then add the oil. Once hot, add the mushrooms, pepper, onion, and a pinch of salt. Cook, stirring often, for 5 minutes. Add the garlic, taco seasoning, and tomato sauce. Stir to combine, then cook, stirring often, for about 1 minute, until the tomato paste has darkened and the spices are fragrant.

2. Lower the heat to medium, then add the tomatoes. Cook for 10 minutes, stirring occasionally, until the tomatoes have thickened and most of the excess liquid has evaporated. Remove from the heat.

3. Preheat the oven to 350°F. Place the tortillas on two baking sheets.

4. Divide the mushroom mixture among the tortillas, then top with the greens and cheese. Bake for about 15 minutes, until the cheese has melted and the tortillas are golden brown and crispy.

5. Serve immediately, topped with the remaining ingredients as desired.

Immune

Kimchi-Mushroom Stew

Korean hot pot soup and stews are so heating and comforting on cold nights. This pungent, spicy version contains both tofu and mushrooms, for contrast and nutrition. I first tried enoki in a dish like this one; a sprig of raw mushrooms was served on top, then stirred in so the residual heat could cook them. This dish is spicy, so if you're trying to clear your sinuses, this could do the trick!

SERVES: 4 | PREP AND COOK TIME: 25 minutes

¼ cup gochugaru (Korean chili powder)

2 tablespoons toasted sesame oil

4 cloves garlic, crushed

2 tablespoons tamari

1 quart (4 cups) mushroom broth

16 ounces soft tofu

1 cup prepared kimchi

2 cups mixed tender mushrooms (oyster, shiitake, and/or enoki)

1 quart (4 cups) water

2 carrots, peeled and julienned

6 cups spinach

4 cups cooked brown rice

4 soft-cooked or poached eggs (optional)

4 scallions, white and green parts, sliced

1. In a small bowl, mix together the gochugaru, sesame oil, garlic, and tamari. Set aside.

2. Combine the broth, tofu, kimchi, mushrooms (except enoki, if using, as they will be added later), and water in large pot. Bring to a boil, then stir in the gochugaru mixture, along with the carrots and spinach. Reduce heat to medium, cover, and simmer for 5 minutes.

3. Divide the brown rice into four bowls, then top with the eggs and enoki mushrooms, if using.

4. Pour the tofu-mushroom mixture over the rice and eggs, then garnish with the scallions.

Immune

Oyster Mushroom Galette with Butternut Squash, Red Onion, and Smoky Pecans

Galettes are rustic French tarts baked on a sheet pan rather than in a pie plate. The edges are folded over to hold in all the tasty ingredients, and they can be sweet or savory. In this one, thinly sliced butternut squash offers a creamy, sweet contrast to tangy onions and rich oyster mushrooms. Don't skip the smoky pecans on top. You'll love their spice and crunch.

SERVES: 4 | PREP AND COOK TIME: 90 minutes

1 small butternut squash (about 1 pound), peeled and thinly sliced

1 pie crust, store-bought or homemade

1 tablespoon fresh thyme

2 tablespoons safflower oil, divided

3 cups oyster mushrooms

1 large red onion, thinly sliced

1 ounce dry sherry

1 tablespoon butter, diced

1 tablespoon thinly sliced fresh sage

4 cups arugula

4 ounces blue cheese or ¼ cup soft almond milk cheese

salt and pepper, to taste

For the pecans:

¼ cup chopped pecans

2 teaspoons maple syrup

½ teaspoon tamari

½ teaspoon smoked paprika

1. Prepare the squash. Preheat the oven to 375°F. Line a baking sheet with parchment paper.

2. Layer the butternut squash on the prepared baking sheet, then sprinkle with the thyme and 1 tablespoon safflower oil, plus salt and pepper. Roast for about 30 minutes, until tender. Let cool. Increase the oven temperature to 400°F.

3. Prepare the mushrooms while the squash is cooking. Place a large skillet over medium-high heat, then add the remaining oil. Once hot, add the oyster mushrooms, onion, and salt. Cook, stirring often, for

5 minutes. Pour in the sherry, then scrape the bottom of the pan to loosen any brown bits. Stir in the sage and remove from the heat.

4. In a small bowl, combine the pecans with the maple syrup, tamari, and smoked paprika.

5. Line a second baking sheet with parchment paper and unroll the pie crust onto the parchment. Leaving a 1-inch border, place one-third of the squash in an overlapping layer. Top with half the mushroom mixture. Layer on another third of the squash, then top with the remaining mushrooms and onions. Finally, add the rest of the squash, then the pecans. Fold in the edges of the crust. Top with the butter and sage.

6. Bake the galette for 30 to 40 minutes, until the crust is cooked through and golden brown.

7. Let cool for 10 minutes, then slice into four wedges. Top each slice with arugula and blue cheese or almond milk cheese.

✚
Cholesterol, Mood, Skin

Savory Pressed Mushroom Hoagies

Pressing mushrooms is a technique that's quite popular these days (hat tip to the Sarno brothers and their site Wicked Healthy Food), and for good reason. This technique maximizes the surface area of the mushroom, so you get more brown, flavor-rich edges. Piled high onto a hoagie bun with loads of other vegetables, this is a two-hands-needed kind of sandwich. A light basil aioli holds everything together.

SERVES: 4 | PREP AND COOK TIME: 30 minutes, plus at least 2 hours to marinate

For the mushrooms:

- 1 tablespoon red miso paste
- 1 tablespoon Worcestershire sauce
- ¼ cup nutritional yeast
- 1 tablespoon Dijon mustard
- 1 tablespoon maple syrup
- ¼ teaspoon black pepper
- 1 tablespoon apple cider vinegar
- 1 tablespoon balsamic vinegar
- 1 tablespoon safflower oil
- 2 tablespoons water
- 4 cups oyster, cremini, or maitake mushrooms, bases trimmed

For the basil aioli:

- 2 tablespoons lemon juice
- ⅛ teaspoon pepper
- ½ cup mayonnaise or silken tofu
- 6 fresh basil leaves

For the sandwiches:

- 4 hoagie rolls
- ½ medium red onion, thinly sliced
- 2 Roma tomatoes, thinly sliced
- 4 cups baby arugula

1. To prepare the mushrooms, combine all ingredients in shallow dish along with 2 tablespoons water. Toss the mushrooms to thoroughly coat. Cover and refrigerate for 2 hours or up to overnight.

2. To prepare the aioli, combine the all ingredients in a blender or mini food processor until smooth. Cover and refrigerate until ready to eat.

3. Once the mushrooms have marinated, preheat the oven to 400°F and position a rack in the middle. Line a baking sheet with parchment paper. Drain the mushrooms, reserving the marinade if desired.

4. Place the mushrooms on the baking sheet in a single layer. Top with another sheet of parchment and a second baking sheet. Place the baking sheets on the middle rack in the oven, then top with a heavy cast-iron skillet or baking dish to weigh everything down.

5. Bake for 30 minutes, flipping the mushrooms halfway through. Baste with additional marinade when you flip them, if desired.

6. To assemble the sandwiches, split open the rolls. Spread on the aioli, then add the mushrooms. Top with the onions, tomato, and arugula.

✚
Immune

Shiitake and Buckwheat with Red Pepper–Miso Sauce

Buckwheat is a cooling grain that's gluten-free, packed with protein, and supportive of the blood sugar. A relative of rhubarb and a staple in Eastern Europe, it has a strong, slightly bitter flavor but a soft texture. In this recipe, you need the roasted variety of buckwheat called kasha, the nutty flavor of which pairs well with sweet and tangy roasted red peppers. Shiitakes are the mushroom of choice for the skin and cholesterol.

SERVES: 4 to 6 | PREP AND COOK TIME: 1 hour

For the buckwheat:

1 tablespoon safflower oil

1 tablespoon butter

1 cup sliced shiitake mushroom caps

2 medium shallots, minced

1 cup toasted buckwheat groats (kasha)

½ teaspoon sweet or smoked paprika

1 ounce dry sherry

½ teaspoon salt

1 ½ cups mushroom broth

For the red pepper miso sauce:

2 whole roasted red peppers, drained and rinsed

1 tablespoon olive oil

1 large clove garlic, minced

½ cup mushroom broth

1 tablespoon red miso paste

1 tablespoon lemon juice

salt and pepper, to taste

1. To prepare the buckwheat, place a large skillet with a lid over medium-high heat. Heat the oil and butter, then add the mushrooms and shallots. Cook, stirring often, for about 5 minutes, until the shiitakes and shallots are soft and starting to get some color. Stir in the buckwheat and the paprika.

2. Add the sherry, then scrape the bottom of the pan to lift any brown bits. Stir in the salt and the broth. Cover and reduce the heat to medium-low. Cook for 18 to 20 minutes, until the buckwheat is tender.

3. While the buckwheat is cooking, prepare the red pepper miso sauce. Puree all the ingredients together until smooth. Season with salt

and pepper to taste. Warm the sauce in a small saucepan set over medium-low heat.

4. Serve the buckwheat and shiitakes with the sauce.

✚
Detox, Cholesterol, Skin

Velvety Tofu with Wood Ear Mushrooms

Both wood ear mushrooms and tofu are yin tonics in TCM, meaning they moisturize conditions of dryness within the body and support bodily fluids. (Appetizing, I know, but it does reinforce that food is medicine.) Wood ears have very little flavor but provide a pleasantly chewy texture. I like to slice them thinly so their texture is evenly dispersed. This dish is a great one for those who claim to dislike either wood ears or tofu; the silky sauce envelopes them both and imparts well-balanced flavor. If you'd like, you can use chicken instead of tofu for this recipe.

SERVES: 4 | PREP AND COOK TIME: 30 minutes

1 pound extra-firm tofu, pressed and cubed

2 tablespoons cornstarch

¼ teaspoon salt

¼ teaspoon pepper

1 tablespoon regular sesame oil

1 ounce dried wood ear mushrooms, soaked in hot water for at least 15 minutes

1 small yellow onion, thinly sliced

1 cup water

1 scallion, white and green parts, sliced

steamed vegetables and cooked brown rice, for serving

For the sauce:

1 tablespoon cornstarch

1 tablespoon toasted sesame oil

1 tablespoon tamari

1 tablespoon red miso paste

3 cloves garlic, minced

1 teaspoon mirin, sake, or rice vinegar

¼ teaspoon crushed red pepper

1. Toss the tofu with the cornstarch, salt and pepper.

2. Place a large skillet or wok over medium-high heat. Add the sesame oil, then add the tofu. Cook until browned on all sides, about 2 minutes per side.

3. Drain the mushrooms and thinly slice them.

4. Add the onions and mushrooms to the pan, and stir to combine.

5. Stir the sauce ingredients together in a small bowl, along with the water. Add to the pan, stir to combine, lower the heat to medium, then cover and let simmer for 10 minutes.

6. Remove from the heat, and serve with steamed vegetables and brown rice.

✚ Cholesterol, Immune, Respiratory System

Tarragon-Thyme Chanterelles with Shallots and Roasted Potatoes

Chanterelles and tarragon are one of my favorite pairings of mushrooms and herbs. A licoricelike, warming herb with a slightly sweet taste, tarragon can quickly overpower a dish, so use less if it is new to you. To me, tarragon is the taste of spring, especially in vinegar- or wine-based sauces like this one. If you're a chanterelle purist, omit the herbs from the mushroom preparation to truly let them shine.

SERVES: 4 | PREP AND COOK TIME: 1 hour

8 potatoes, cut into 1-inch cubes

1 tablespoon safflower oil

1 teaspoon fresh thyme

zest and juice of 1 lemon

2 tablespoons olive oil

1 large shallot, minced

1 pound chanterelle mushrooms, wiped clean and chopped

1 teaspoon fresh thyme

1 teaspoon fresh tarragon, minced

½ cup dry white wine

1 tablespoon butter

salt and pepper, to taste

1. Preheat the oven to 425°F. Line a baking sheet with parchment paper.

2. Toss the potatoes with the safflower oil, thyme, and lemon juice, then season with salt and pepper. Transfer to the prepared baking sheet. Roast for about 40 minutes, until browned and fork-tender.

3. Meanwhile, heat the olive oil in a medium skillet over medium-high heat. Add the shallot and sauté, stirring often, until it starts to turn color, about 5 minutes. Add the chanterelles and cook for about 5 minutes more, until the mushrooms are cooked through. Stir in the thyme and tarragon, then deglaze the pan with the wine, scraping up any brown bits from the bottom of the pan. Stir in the butter. Remove from the heat and season to taste with salt and pepper.

4. Before serving, toss the potatoes with the lemon zest, then divide among four plates. Top with the chanterelles.

✚ Cardiovascular, Detox, Immune

Mushroom Paprikash

This is a slight variation on the comfort food my mom served up throughout my childhood. Paprika's sweet, smoky, and sometimes spicy notes are delightful with mushrooms, and any tender mushroom will do in this recipe. Don't rush the tomato paste and paprikas as they cook down; they'll develop such flavor from this step. To make the dish gluten-free, swap out the flour for 1 teaspoon cornstarch.

SERVES: 4 | PREP AND COOK TIME: 40 minutes

1 tablespoon butter

1 tablespoon olive oil

1 large yellow onion, thinly sliced

1 leek, white parts only, sliced

1 pound mushrooms (cremini, oyster, and/or maitake)

1 pound chicken or seitan, cut into bite-size pieces, or 1 (14.5-ounce) can chickpeas

1 tablespoon tomato paste

2 tablespoons sweet paprika

1 tablespoon smoked paprika

pinch of crushed red pepper

3 cloves garlic, minced

2 tablespoons whole-wheat, pastry, or all-purpose flour

1 (14.5-ounce) can diced tomatoes

½ cup sour cream or unsweetened cashew yogurt

chopped fresh flat-leaf parsley, for garnish

4 servings polenta, prepared according to package directions, for serving

salt and pepper, to taste

1. Heat a large skillet over medium-high heat. Add the butter and oil, and when the butter melts, add the onion and leeks. Sauté, stirring often, for about 5 minutes, until they start to soften and take on color. Add the mushrooms and desired protein, and cook another 5 minutes, stirring often.

2. Lower the heat to medium. Stir in the tomato paste, sweet and smoked paprika, crushed red pepper, garlic, and flour, and cook until the tomato paste and paprikas are darkened and fragrant, about 2 minutes.

3. Add the tomatoes, then refill the can with water and add that too. Reduce heat to low, cover, and cook for 10 minutes, until the sauce is bubbly.

4. Remove from heat and stir in the sour cream or cashew yogurt. Season with salt and pepper to taste. Divide the polenta among four bowls, then top with the paprikash. Sprinkle with parsley and serve immediately.

✚ Immune

Sea to Shore Salad

This salad was inspired by one I had on my honeymoon in Vancouver, and I tried my best to re-create it at home. It can stand alone as a meal, and it's a feast for the eyes. Don't let the number of ingredients and steps intimidate you; the process is quite simple, and the result is a hearty yet light, filling bowl that celebrates the bounty of nature—mushrooms and plants from both sea and shore.

SERVES: 4 | PREP AND COOK TIME: 1 hour

For the dressing:

- 1 carrot, peeled and roughly chopped
- 2 tablespoons white or chickpea miso paste
- 1 teaspoon grated fresh ginger
- ¼ cup tahini
- 1 teaspoon tamari
- 1 clove garlic
- ½ cup water

For the mushrooms:

- 1 teaspoon safflower or regular sesame oil
- 1 cup sliced shiitake mushrooms (caps only)
- 1 teaspoon toasted sesame oil
- ½ teaspoon tamari
- pinch of crushed red pepper

For the salad:

- ¼ cup rice vinegar
- 2 tablespoons mirin
- 1 tablespoon tamari
- 4 cups shredded purple cabbage
- 1 bunch kale, leaves only, chopped
- 1 cup mixed dried seaweed, soaked in water for at least 30 minutes
- 1 cup quinoa
- 1 teaspoon ground turmeric
- 1 teaspoon grated fresh ginger
- ¼ teaspoon black pepper
- 1 cup sliced or shredded daikon
- 4 scallions, white and green parts, sliced
- 1 large carrot, peeled and shredded
- 1 cup mixed sprouts
- ¼ cup chopped cilantro
- 1 avocado, sliced or diced
- 4 teaspoons toasted sesame seeds

1. To prepare the dressing, blend all the ingredients together in a blender or mini food processor. Once smooth, transfer to a jar and set aside. (Dressing can be made up to one day in advance.)

2. To prepare the mushrooms, heat the oil in small skillet over medium heat. Add the shiitakes and cook, stirring often, for about 4 minutes, until they soften and darken. Stir in the toasted sesame oil, tamari, and red pepper. Remove from heat and set aside.

3. To prepare the salads, combine the rice vinegar, mirin, and tamari in a small bowl.

4. Place the cabbage and kale in a large bowl, and add half the vinegar mixture. Massage until shiny and slightly softened. Set aside.

5. Drain the sea vegetables, then toss with the remaining dressing. Set aside.

6. Prepare the quinoa according to package directions, adding the turmeric, ginger, and black pepper to the pot as it cooks.

7. To assemble the salads, divide the cabbage and kale, quinoa, sea vegetables, and mushrooms among four bowls. I like to make decorative piles of each ingredient. Divide the daikon, scallions, carrots, sprouts, cilantro, and avocado among the bowls. Serve with the dressing and garnish with the sesame seeds.

✚ Cholesterol, Detox, Immune, Skin

Creamy Old Bay King Oyster "Scallops"

When marinated in classic Old Bay seasoning and sliced into hearty rounds, king oyster mushrooms are a pretty convincing stand-in for scallops—especially once they've been seared and braised. Corn gives the dish a bit more heft, while artichokes lend their lightness and detoxifying properties.

SERVES: 4 | PREP AND COOK TIME: 2 hours, 15 minutes

For the marinade:

1 teaspoon kelp seasoning blend

2 teaspoons Old Bay seasoning blend

2 tablespoons safflower oil or melted butter

1 tablespoon lemon juice

1 tablespoon apple cider vinegar

⅛ teaspoon pepper

For the "scallops":

2 (6-ounce) packages king oyster mushrooms, sliced into ¾-inch rounds

1 tablespoon safflower oil

2 cloves garlic, minced

1 cup artichoke hearts

1 cup corn kernels (optional)

½ cup dry white wine

1 tablespoon butter

1 tablespoon heavy cream or cashew cream

1 tablespoon chopped flat-leaf parsley, for garnish

prepared mashed potatoes or grits, for serving

1. Mix all marinade ingredients together in a container with a tight-fitting lid. Add the mushrooms, toss to combine, and marinate for at least 2 hours. Remove the mushrooms and reserve the remaining marinade.

2. Place a large skillet over medium-high heat. Add the oil, then sear the mushrooms on both sides, about two minutes per side, then add the remaining marinade, garlic, artichoke hearts, and corn, if using. Deglaze the pan with the wine, scraping the bottom to loosen any brown bits.

3. Reduce the heat to medium-low. Cover and cook for 10 minutes, until the sauce has thickened and artichokes and corn are heated through

4. Stir in the butter and cream. Serve immediately, topped with the parsley, over mashed potatoes or grits.

✚ Cholesterol, Immune

CHAPTER 7

Snacks

This chapter is diverse—you'll find snacks that are sweet and savory, with both tough and tender mushrooms. The recipes were developed with specific purposes in mind. Some include additional herbal adaptogens for energy or stress support, while others simply add a powdered extract to a familiar snack, like granola or kale chips. If you're interested in taking a specific mushroom powder on a regular basis, you might find inspiration in this chapter.

Adaptogen Energy Balls

These energy balls are a staple in my house, and I've shared them with my yoga students enough times that they request them for special events. A fellow teacher who's in acupuncture school makes them before big tests. This version is always with me when I travel, to help combat stress. Use any adaptogens you like. I like licorice because it is sweet and also has traditionally been used to help the body regulate cortisol (and studies back that up).[60] Ginseng is a stimulating adaptogen without making me jittery like caffeine does, as is eleuthero. Goji berries are actually adaptogenic and used to build energy in TCM. Of course, I add cordyceps and reishi too.

MAKES: 16 | PREP TIME: 20 minutes

1 cup almonds

1 cup pitted dates, soaked in hot water for 10 minutes then drained

½ cup goji berries

1 serving powdered cordyceps extract

1 serving powdered reishi extract

2 droppers licorice root tincture

1 teaspoon ground eleuthero

1 teaspoon ashwagandha powder

½ teaspoon ground ginseng

pinch of sea salt

2 tablespoons unsweetened shredded coconut

2 tablespoons hemp hearts

1. Pulse the almonds in a food processor until coarsely ground. Transfer to a medium bowl.

2. Pulse the dates with the goji berries, cordyceps and reishi extracts, licorice, eleuthero, ashwagandha, ginseng, and salt until a thick paste forms. Add the almonds and pulse until the mixture is thoroughly combined.

3. Mix together the coconut and hemp hearts in the bowl that held the almonds.

4. Wet your hands and form the almond-date mixture into table-spoon-size balls. Roll in the coconut-hemp mixture.

5. Refrigerate for up to 1 week or eat immediately.

✚
Energy, Immune, Mood, Stress

Stress-Relieving Smoothie

Smoothies are a stress reliever in and of themselves—you can have a nutritious, filling snack or meal in mere minutes with little mess. I included some of my favorite stress-busting foods in this one. Hemp lends omega-3s, blueberries support the memory, and cacao's flavonoids help the brain in numerous ways.[61] Avocado ensures your smoothie is creamy and rich, with plenty of heart-healthy fats.

SERVES: 1 | PREP TIME: 5 minutes

1 cup oat milk or another milk

1 cup blueberries

1 tablespoon raw cacao powder or dark cocoa powder

½ avocado

3 tablespoons hemp seeds

1 serving powdered reishi extract

Combine all the ingredients in a blender and process until smooth, adding water to thin it if desired. Drink immediately.

✚ Adaptogenic, Immune, Memory, Stress, Sleep

The "I Overdid It" Detox Smoothie

Whether you overdid it on booze, food, or some combination of the two, put this smoothie on the menu as soon as you can. It's potent, with maitake and shiitake to support detox and the immune system, plenty of vitamin C, and other antioxidants. I included pineapple, turmeric, and ginger for their anti-inflammatory properties, plus moringa, a superfood green with more iron than spinach, more potassium than bananas, and more vitamin C than oranges![62]

SERVES: 1 | PREP TIME: 5 minutes

1 cup fresh or frozen pineapple chunks

1 cup dandelion greens

1 cup kale

1 medium grapefruit, peeled, segmented, and seeded

¼ cup unsweetened cranberry juice

1-inch piece fresh ginger

2 tablespoons lime juice

1 tablespoon moringa powder

1 serving powdered shiitake extract

1 serving powdered maitake extract

½ teaspoon ground turmeric

Combine all the ingredients in a blender and process until smooth, adding water to thin it if desired. Drink immediately.

✚ Detox, Immune

Supergreen Detox Smoothie

The name says it all: This smoothie is super green, and it's intended to support our natural detox processes. It won't be a smoothie you crave for its flavor, but it does pack a bright green punch. Chlorella is a single-cell green algae that provides chlorophyll and numerous nutrients, while spirulina is a single-cell blue-green algae that is also touted for its nutrition, including protein content. I also included moringa, whose notable nutrition contributions include iron, potassium, and vitamin C. Banana and coconut offer creaminess and palatability, but if the flavor is still too strong for you, feel free to add ginger.

SERVES: 1 | PREP TIME: 2 minutes

1 cup almond milk

½ cup frozen young coconut pieces

1 serving powdered shiitake extract

1 medium banana

1 teaspoon chlorella

1 teaspoon spirulina

1 tablespoon moringa powder

1 cup spinach or kale

Combine all the ingredients in a blender and process until smooth, adding water to thin it if desired. Drink immediately.

✚ Antioxidant, Detox, Immune

Beauty Smoothie

This smoothie is carefully curated. While it is delicious, I chose the ingredients more for their nutrition than flavor. Rosehips are rich in vitamin C, as are moringa and currants, and we need this antioxidant for collagen production and immune support. Cucumber provides silica, a mineral that supports healthy connective tissues and the skin. Flax and hemp offer omega-3s—these essential fatty acids support the skin as well as the heart and brain.[63] Of course, chaga offers antioxidants, while shiitake is there for the skin and liver, which as our primary detox organ also supports healthy skin.

SERVES: 1 | PREP TIME: 5 minutes

1 tablespoon ground flaxseed

2 tablespoons hemp hearts

1 tablespoon dried currants

½ cup prepared iced rosehip tea

½ cup prepared iced green tea

1 serving powdered shiitake extract

1 serving powdered chaga extract

½ medium cucumber

1 tablespoon moringa powder

½ avocado

1 orange, peeled, segmented, and seeded

Combine all the ingredients in a blender and process until smooth, adding water to thin it if desired. Drink immediately.

Beauty, Detox, Immune

Blood-Builder Smoothie

In Western medicine and nutrition, we don't talk much about building the blood, but it's commonly discussed in TCM and other traditional forms of medicine. I called this smoothie a blood builder because I included beets, which help oxygen uptake of blood, as well as molasses, which has high amounts of iron. The dates naturally sweeten this smoothie and add more iron.

SERVES: 1 | PREP TIME: 10 minutes

1 cup milk

2 pitted dates

1 banana

1 tablespoon beet powder or 1 small cooked beet (with no added seasonings)

1 teaspoon chaga

1 serving powdered maitake extract

1 tablespoon blackstrap molasses

Combine all the ingredients in a blender and process until smooth, adding water to thin it if desired. Drink immediately.

✚ Antioxidant, Energy, Immune

Immune-Boosting Smoothie

When we're sick, we often crave comfort food, but we really should be choosing simple, easy-to-digest foods packed with the nutrients our immune system needs. Enter this smoothie, which I sip throughout fall and winter whether I feel right as rain or under the weather. Black elderberry is a powerhouse of antioxidants, as is chaga, and I include turmeric and ginger for inflammation. Drinkable yogurt (I opt for cashew kefir) provides probiotics to help the immune system via the gut and gives this smoothie a tangy taste.

SERVES: 1 | PREP TIME: 5 minutes

1 teaspoon black elderberry syrup

1 serving powdered chaga extract

½ serving powdered maitake extract

½ serving powdered reishi extract

1 cup drinkable yogurt with active cultures

3 cups baby spinach

1 small banana

½ teaspoon grated fresh ginger

½ teaspoon grated fresh or ground turmeric

Combine all the ingredients in a blender and process until smooth, adding water to thin it if desired. Drink immediately.

✚ Adaptogenic, Antioxidant, Blood Sugar, Immune, Sleep, Stress

Blueberry-Lavender-Cacao Memory Smoothie

I attend an herbal conference outside Asheville every summer, and a couple of years ago, everyone was buzzing about berries. As it turns out, they're excellent for the brain, especially as we age.[64] I eat a ½ cup every day for their antioxidant support and deliciousness. They take center stage in this smoothie, which also includes lion's mane and cordyceps. I added plenty of cacao, which also enhances cognition.[65] Lavender is fragrant and naturally calming, so I added a bit of that as well.

SERVES: 1 | PREP TIME: 5 minutes

¼ cup old-fashioned oats

1 cup soymilk

1 scoop vanilla or plain protein powder (optional)

1 serving powdered lion's mane extract

1 serving powdered cordyceps extract

1 cup blueberries

2 tablespoons raw cacao or dark cocoa powder

pinch of vanilla powder

pinch of dried lavender

Combine all the ingredients in a blender and process until smooth, adding water to thin it if desired. Drink immediately.

✚ Energy, Immune, Memory

Cherry-Chaga Cheesecake Smoothie

Confession: I made this smoothie because I liked the name. Turns out, the flavor combination really works. While cheesecake filling may be delicious enough to drink, it doesn't exactly jibe with the theme of this smoothie, so I created a creamy, tangy cheesecake taste with cashews, coconut milk, and lemon juice, plus vanilla and a little maple syrup. The cherries are, well, the cherry on top (and tart cherries support recovery from endurance exercise, so feel free to swap those in)![66]

SERVES: 1 | PREP TIME: 5 minutes

1 cup coconut milk

2 tablespoons raw cashews

1 scoop vanilla or plain protein powder (optional)

1 tablespoon lemon juice

1 cup frozen cherries

1 serving powdered chaga extract

pinch of vanilla powder or ¼ teaspoon vanilla extract

1 teaspoon maple syrup or honey

Combine all the ingredients in a blender and process until smooth, adding water to thin it if desired. Drink immediately.

✚ Antioxidant, Immune,

Pomegranate-Aloe Beauty Spritzer

As with the Beauty Smoothie (page 141), this spritzer was carefully developed based on the properties of each ingredient. Turkey tail supports bones, joints, and the skin, while reishi is included for its adaptogenic qualities. Shiitake promotes healthy skin and natural detox functions. Aloe vera might be familiar to you as a topical skin treatment, but it also supports skin from the inside out. Pomegranate is bursting with antioxidants, so I used that as the base.

SERVES: 1 | PREP TIME: 5 minutes

4 leaves fresh mint

½ serving turkey tail mushroom tincture

½ serving reishi mushroom tincture

½ serving shiitake mushroom tincture

1 cup pomegranate juice

¼ cup aloe vera juice

sparkling water, to top

Tear the mint leaves and place them in a glass. Fill the glass with ice, then add the turkey tail, reishi, and shiitake tinctures and the pomegranate and aloe vera juices. Stir to combine, then top with sparkling water. Serve immediately.

✚ Adaptogenic, Beauty, Detox, Immune

Mango Lassi with Turmeric and Cordyceps

When I stopped eating dairy, I missed the creamy lassis I ordered when going out for Indian food. I started making my own once non-dairy kefir became easy to find. This lassi is designed for recovery from a long workout, as I daydreamed about it on a run. The protein powder is optional, but don't skip the maca—like cordyceps, it is an adaptogen that provides energy.

SERVES: 1 | PREP TIME: 5 minutes

1 cup dairy or non-dairy kefir

1 scoop vanilla or plain protein powder (optional)

1 serving powdered cordyceps extract

1 teaspoon maca powder

2 pitted dates

1 cup fresh or frozen mango chunks

½ teaspoon ground turmeric

½ teaspoon grated fresh ginger

¼ teaspoon ground cardamom

Combine all the ingredients in a blender and process until smooth. Serve immediately.

✚ Adaptogenic, Energy, Immune, Stress

'Shroom and Nootch Popcorn

Air-popped popcorn is a more nutritious alternative to chips when you're craving something crunchy. Savory mushroom powders blend right in, and you can't been the cheesy, umami-filled flavor of nutritional yeast ("nootch") on popcorn. I always make sure my corn—fresh, frozen, or dried for popping—is non-GMO.

SERVES: 4 | PREP AND COOK TIME: 10 minutes

1 serving powdered reishi extract

¼ cup nutritional yeast

¼ teaspoon ground turmeric

½ teaspoon smoked paprika or curry powder

12 cups air-popped popcorn

2 tablespoons melted ghee or coconut oil

salt and pepper, to taste

1. Combine the reishi extract, nutritional yeast, turmeric, and smoked paprika or curry in a small bowl.

2. Place the popcorn in a large bowl, preferably one with a lid. (I use a Pyrex mixing bowl for this.)

3. Drizzle on the ghee or coconut oil, then sprinkle on the spice blend. Season with salt and pepper, put the lid on, and give it a good shake. Serve immediately.

✚ Immune

Mushroom Hummus

This is more of a chickpea-mushroom dip than a traditional hummus, but it's tasty nonetheless. Balsamic brings a sweet tanginess, which I find to be a lovely way to join chickpeas and mushrooms. Don't rush the pureeing process. There's something so decadent about velvety smooth hummus. (This is, no surprise, a great recipe for those who dislike the texture of mushrooms.)

SERVES: 4 to 6 | PREP AND COOK TIME: 20 minutes

1 tablespoon safflower oil

1 cup mixed mushrooms, finely diced (shiitake, maitake, etc.)

1 medium red onion, thinly sliced

2 (14.5-ounce) cans chickpeas, drained and rinsed, or 3 cups cooked chickpeas

juice of 1 lemon

¼ cup balsamic vinegar

1 teaspoon salt, plus more to taste

2 tablespoons olive oil

2 tablespoons tahini

½ cup water

crushed red pepper, for garnish

olive oil, for garnish

minced flat-leaf parsley, for garnish

salt and black pepper, to taste

1. Place a medium skillet over medium-high heat. Once hot, add the oil, then the mushrooms and onion. Sauté for 5 to 7 minutes, until the mushrooms are golden brown. Season to taste with salt and pepper. Reserve 1 tablespoon for garnish and transfer the rest of the mushroom-onion mixture to a blender.

2. Add the chickpeas, lemon juice, vinegar, 1 teaspoon salt, olive oil, and tahini to the blender, blend until smooth, then stream in the water to achieve the desired consistency. The hummus should be smooth and fluffy. Season to taste with salt and pepper.

3. Transfer to a bowl and garnish with the reserved mushrooms, crushed red pepper, olive oil, and parsley.

✚ Immune

Coconut-Cashew Mushroom-Matcha Butter

I first discovered matcha as a culinary ingredient in Seoul. Beyond its myriad uses in tea drinks, I enjoyed it in pastries, candy (green tea Kit Kats!), and even gum. My love of all things green tea has endured, for both the gentle caffeine buzz and antioxidant protection. I love mixing matcha with rich, fatty ingredients like coconut and nuts. I eat this cashew-coconut butter straight up with a spoon and on bananas. Due to the coconut oil, it will firm up in the fridge, so bring it to room temperature before spreading. For an extra treat, roll the butter into balls and drizzle with bittersweet chocolate.

MAKES: about 1 cup | PREP TIME: 10 minutes

½ cup cashews

1 tablespoon coconut oil

½ cup unsweetened shredded coconut

2 teaspoons matcha powder

1 serving powdered cordyceps extract

1 serving powdered chaga extract

¼ teaspoon vanilla powder

1 teaspoon coconut sugar

pinch of sea salt

1. Blend the cashews in a mini food processor until smooth and creamy. Add the coconut oil and pulse to combine, then add the remaining ingredients. Process until it reaches the desired consistency.

2. Transfer to a sealed jar and refrigerate for up to 1 week.

✚ Energy, Immune, Stress

Reishi Mixed Nut Butter

The combination of walnuts, almonds, and pecans creates a unique nut butter that's slightly sweet, allowing the reishi to blend right in. Feel free to adjust the nuts based on what you have on hand—I've experimented with sunflower, sesame, and pumpkin seeds too. Try it on cinnamon-raisin bread or sweet potato toast.

MAKES: 1½ cups | PREP TIME: 10 minutes

½ cup walnuts

½ cup pecans

½ cup almonds

1 tablespoon safflower or coconut oil

2 tablespoons powdered reishi extract

sea salt, to taste

Blend all ingredients together in a mini food processor until smooth. Transfer to a sealed jar and refrigerate for up to 1 week.

✚ Adaptogenic, Immune, Sleep, Stress

Nutty Coconut Mushroom Granola

This is the granola of my dreams: sweet, crunchy, and slightly clumpy with a hint of salt. I load up on the good stuff—nuts, seeds, and dried fruit (and mushrooms)—for a filling, tasty topping to the cashew yogurt and blueberry parfaits I eat most afternoons. This makes a huge batch, enough for two of us to eat it daily for two weeks or so.

MAKES: about 4 cups | PREP AND COOK TIME: 1 hour, 15 minutes

3 tablespoons coconut oil

1/3 cup maple syrup

2 tablespoons coconut or raw sugar

1/3 cup canned coconut milk

3/4 teaspoon sea salt

1 teaspoon vanilla extract

3 cups old-fashioned oats

1/2 cup unsweetened coconut flakes

6 servings powdered mushroom extract (any variety)

1 teaspoon ground cinnamon

1/2 cup chopped nuts

1/2 cup hemp hearts, sesame, chia, and ground flaxseed

1. Preheat the oven to 325°F. Line two baking sheets with parchment paper.

2. Place a small saucepan over medium heat. Add the coconut oil, maple syrup, coconut or raw sugar, coconut milk, salt, and vanilla. Simmer until the sugar dissolves.

3. Grind half the oats in a food processor.

4. Transfer the ground nuts to a large bowl along with the remaining oats, coconut flakes, mushroom powder, cinnamon, and nuts. Pour the maple syrup mixture over the oats. Stir to combine.

5. Divide between the prepared baking sheets.

6. Bake for about 45 minutes, turning the mixture halfway through. The granola is done when it starts to get crispy and is evenly golden

brown. Immediately sprinkle on the seeds. Let cool completely, then transfer to a sealed container and store for up to 1 month.

✚ Immune

Umami-Laced Kale Chips

Kale chips are addictively delicious, thanks to this salty, tangy coating. Adding mushroom powder not only gives them extra immune support, it also gives them extra umami. These taste somewhat like nacho tortilla chips, thanks to the vinegar and nutritional yeast. If you struggle to eat kale, try it this way!

SERVES: 2 to 4 | PREP AND COOK TIME: 30 minutes

¼ cup tahini

2 tablespoons tamari

2 tablespoons apple cider vinegar

⅓ cup nutritional yeast

1 teaspoon ground cumin

½ teaspoon smoked paprika

¼ teaspoon crushed red pepper (optional)

2 cloves garlic, minced or pressed

3 servings powdered turkey tail extract

3 servings powdered maitake extract

2 bunches kale, stems removed

1. Preheat the oven to 350°F. Line two baking sheets with parchment paper.

2. Combine all the ingredients except the kale in a blender and process until smooth.

3. Transfer the mixture to a bowl, then add 3 tablespoons of water to the blender. Pulse to "clean out" the blender, and add this water to the bowl. Add the kale, then use your hands to thoroughly coat each piece.

4. Place the kale in a single layer on the prepared baking sheets.

5. Bake for 15 to 20 minutes, until the kale is crispy.

6. Remove from the oven, allow to cool, then eat immediately. Kale can be stored for up to 2 days in an air-tight container, but this snack is best when fresh.

✚ Immune

No-Bake Mushroom Granola Bites

These granola bites are small and chewy, which is how I prefer my granola bars. They're another common snack at my house, and I change up the mushroom powders based on what's going on in our lives. If it's winter, I lean toward chaga and turkey tail; if we're super busy, I reach for reishi and cordyceps. While writing this book, I put lion's mane into everything I could!

MAKES: 16 | PREP AND COOK TIME: 20 minutes, plus 2 hours to chill

½ cup chopped nuts

½ cup creamy nut butter

3 cups old-fashioned oats

1 cup maple syrup

½ cup dried fruit

¼ cup hemp hearts

¼ cup chia seeds

½ teaspoon salt

1 teaspoon ground cinnamon

1 teaspoon vanilla extract

6 servings powdered mushroom extract, any variety

1. Place a large saucepan over medium heat. Add all ingredients, and stir well to combine. Cook, stirring often, until the mixture is thoroughly combined.

2. Line a 9 x 13-inch pan with parchment paper. Transfer the mixture to the pan, and pat down firmly and evenly with a wet offset spatula.

3. Allow to cool completely or refrigerate for 2 hours before slicing. Store in an air-tight container for up to 1 week.

✚ Immune

Carob-Chaga Bites

My mother once played a dirty trick on my sister and me. She served us carob cookies and called them chocolate chip cookies. Carob is not chocolate. If you set out believing it is just like chocolate, you will be disappointed, as I was. As an adult, I rediscovered carob and have quite an affinity for it. Carob, which comes from the pods of the locust tree, is caffeine-free and sweet, with three times the calcium as cocoa.[67] I especially love the combination of carob and chaga, which play nicely off each other in these sweet bites.

MAKES: 16 | PREP TIME: 15 minutes

1 cup almonds

1½ cups pitted dates, soaked in hot water for at least 10 minutes and drained well

¼ cup carob powder

2 servings powdered chaga extract

pinch of sea salt

almond meal, as needed

1. Place the almonds in a food processor. Pulse until roughly chopped, then transfer to a medium bowl.

2. Add the dates to the food processor and pulse several times, then add the carob powder, chaga extract, and sea salt and process until a large ball forms.

3. Transfer the date mixture to the bowl with the nuts, and use your hands or a sturdy wooden spoon to combine.

4. Place a sheet of parchment paper on your work surface and turn the "dough" onto it. Using the parchment to keep your hands clean, press the dough into a 1-inch thick rectangle. If the dough seems sticky, sprinkle with a bit of almond meal. Slice into 16 bites or roll into balls.

5. Store in a sealed container in the refrigerator for up to 1 week.

✚ Antioxidant, Immune

Cordyceps-Ashwagandha Energy Bites

These bites are for the athletes out there. I make a batch for long hikes or for snacks when I'm training for races. Since beets are a superfood that can aid athletes with increased oxygen uptake, I added some beet powder, plus orange zest for vitamin C and flavor (to mask the earthy beet taste if you're sensitive to it). Dates are my favorite source of carbs on long runs, since they taste like caramel. Here, they naturally sweeten and bind these bites.

MAKES: 16 | PREP TIME: 20 minutes

1 cup almonds

1 cup pitted dates, soaked in hot water for at least 10 minutes and drained well

¼ cup old-fashioned oats

1 tablespoon beet powder

3 servings powdered cordyceps extract

1 tablespoon ashwagandha powder

zest of 1 orange

¼ cup orange juice

pinch of sea salt

almond meal, as needed

1. Place the almonds in a food processor. Pulse until roughly chopped, then transfer to a medium bowl.

2. Add the dates to the food processor and pulse several times, then add the remaining ingredients and process until a large ball forms.

3. Transfer the date mixture to the bowl with the nuts, and use your hands or a sturdy wooden spoon to combine.

4. Place a sheet of parchment paper on your work surface and turn the "dough" onto it. Using the parchment to keep your hands clean, press the dough into a 1-inch thick rectangle. If the dough seems sticky, sprinkle with a bit of almond meal. Slice into 16 bites or roll into balls.

5. Store in a sealed container in the refrigerator for up to 1 week.

✚
Energy, Immune, Stress

Stress-Busting Energy Bites

These little two-bite snacks are the perfect pick-me-up. I make up a batch every few days, depending on my mood and what kind of support my mind and body needs. I also included my three favorite herbs for stress and mood: holy basil (keeps you centered when you feel like the world is spinning around you); passionflower (my absolute favorite for soothing the nervous system); and lemon balm (gently calms nervous minds and bellies). When I'm too keyed up to eat before a big event, I pack some of these to take the edge off my nerves and hunger.

MAKES: 16 | PREP TIME: 20 minutes

½ cup almonds

¼ cup walnuts

¼ cup old-fashioned oats

1 cup pitted dates, soaked in hot water for at least 10 minutes and drained well

½ cup dried pineapple, finely chopped

1 serving powdered reishi extract

1 serving powdered cordyceps extract

1 serving powdered turkey tail extract

2 droppers passionflower tincture

2 droppers holy basil tincture

2 droppers lemon balm tincture

1 teaspoon lemon zest

pinch of sea salt

¼ cup hemp hearts

1. Place the almonds, walnuts, and oats in a food processor. Pulse until roughly chopped, then transfer to a medium bowl.

2. Add the dates to the food processor and pulse several times, then add the remaining ingredients, except the hemp hearts, and process until a large ball forms.

3. Transfer the date mixture to the bowl with the nuts, and use your hands or a sturdy wooden spoon to combine.

4. Place a sheet of parchment paper on your work surface, and turn the "dough" onto it. Using the parchment to keep your hands clean, press the dough into a 1-inch thick rectangle. Sprinkle the hemp hearts on both sides. Slice into 16 bites or roll into balls.

5. Store in a sealed container in the refrigerator for up to one week.

✚ Adaptogenic, Energy, Immune, Sleep, Stress

Immune-Season Energy Bites

I have a multi-faceted approach to immune support. In addition to washing hands, getting plenty of sleep, and trying to manage stress, I use herbs offensively and defensively. I diffuse and inhale them. I take them in capsule, tincture, and tea form. And I eat them. Vitamin C is necessary for production of cortisol (a "stress hormone"), and it's also crucial for immune health. These bites help me squeeze in plenty of it, thanks to the cranberries and especially the currants. I love spicy ginger for its ability to clear my sinuses and offer antioxidant and anti-inflammatory support. And, of course, I used mushrooms—turkey tail and chaga, but you can use any of the major immune-boosters.

MAKES: 16 | PREP TIME: 20 minutes

½ cup almonds

½ cup pecans

1 cup pitted dates, soaked in hot water for at least 10 minutes and drained well

½ cup dried cranberries

¼ cup candied ginger

1 tablespoon currants

½ cup old-fashioned oats

zest of 1 orange

1 serving powdered turkey tail extract

1 serving powdered chaga extract

pinch of sea salt

¼ cup hemp hearts, for topping

1. Place the almonds and pecans in a food processor. Pulse until roughly chopped, then transfer to a medium bowl.

2. Add the dates, cranberries, currants, and ginger, and pulse several times, then add the orange zest, turkey tail and chaga extracts, and salt, and process until a large ball forms.

3. Transfer the date mixture to the bowl with the nuts, and use your hands or a sturdy wooden spoon to combine.

4. Place a sheet of parchment paper on your work surface and turn the "dough" onto it. Using the parchment to keep your hands clean, press the dough into a 1-inch thick rectangle. Sprinkle the hemp hearts on both sides. Slice into 16 bites.

5. Store in a sealed container in the refrigerator for up to one week.

Immune

Memory Bites

These bites are my favorite snack when I'm giving presentations or teaching more than usual. I used blueberries mostly for flavor, though they do support the brain, plus plenty of cocoa powder for brain health (and because chocolate). On the herbal side, I reached for holy basil (since stress impacts memory) and peppermint, which is stimulating. I opted for the adaptogenic combo of cordyceps and reishi, as well as lion's mane, but you can always adjust based on your tastes.

MAKES: 16 | PREP TIME: 20 minutes

1 cup almonds

½ cup hemp hearts, divided

1½ cups pitted dates, soaked in hot water for at least 10 minutes and drained well

½ cup dried blueberries, soaked in hot water for at least 10 minutes and drained well

¼ cup raw cacao powder or dark cocoa powder

4 droppers holy basil tincture

4 droppers peppermint tincture or ¼ teaspoon peppermint extract

3 servings powdered lion's mane extract

1 serving powdered cordyceps extract

1 serving powdered reishi extract

pinch of sea salt

1. Place almonds and ¼ cup of the hemp hearts in a food processor. Pulse until roughly chopped, then transfer to a medium bowl. Add the dates to the food processor and pulse several times, then add the remaining ingredients and process until a large ball forms.

2. Transfer the date mixture to the bowl with the nuts, and use your hands or a sturdy wooden spoon to combine.

3. Place a sheet of parchment paper on your work surface and turn the "dough" onto it. Using the parchment to keep your hands clean, press the dough into a 1-inch thick rectangle. Sprinkle the remaining hemp hearts on both sides. Slice into 16 bites.

4. Store in a sealed container in the refrigerator for up to 1 week.

➕ Adaptogenic, Immune, Memory, Nervous System, Stress

Energy Bites for Athletes

These are similar to the Cordyceps-Ashwagandha Energy Bites (page 157), but with more of a boost—including more beet powder. I opted to add maca, which is a stimulating and energizing adaptogen. And the tart cherries may help with recovery!

MAKES: 16 | PREP TIME: 20 minutes

1 cup almonds

¾ cup dried tart cherries

¾ cup pitted dates, soaked in hot water for at least 10 minutes and drained well

1 tablespoon maca powder

3 servings powdered cordyceps extract

2 tablespoons beet powder

1 tablespoon orange zest

pinch of sea salt

¼ cup hemp hearts

1. Place the almonds in a food processor. Pulse until roughly chopped, then transfer to a medium bowl.

2. Add the dates to and pulse several times, then add the remaining ingredients and process until a large ball forms.

3. Transfer the date mixture to the bowl with the nuts, and use your hands or a sturdy wooden spoon to combine.

4. Place a sheet of parchment paper on your work surface and turn the "dough" onto it. Using the parchment to keep your hands clean, press the dough into a 1-inch thick rectangle. Sprinkle the hemp hearts on both sides. Slice into 16 bites.

5. Store in a sealed container in the refrigerator for up to 1 week.

✚ Energy, Immune

Beauty Bites

With these bites, the emphasis is on the omega-3s in the form of hemp, chia, and flaxseeds, which pair well with vitamin C and antioxidant-rich superfruits. Since these are beauty bites, shiitake is my mushroom of choice, plus chaga for more antioxidants.

MAKES: 16 | PREP TIME: 20 minutes

½ cup almonds

½ cup hemp hearts, divided

2 tablespoons chia seeds

2 tablespoons ground flaxseed

1½ cups pitted dates, soaked in hot water for at least 10 minutes and drained well

zest of 1 orange

2 tablespoons acai or pomegranate powder

2 servings powdered shiitake extract

1 serving powdered chaga extract

1. Place the almonds and ¼ cup of the hemp hearts in a food processor. Pulse until roughly chopped, then transfer to a medium bowl.

2. Add the dates to the food processor and pulse several times, then add the remaining ingredients and process until a large ball forms.

3. Transfer the date mixture to the bowl with the nuts, and use your hands or a sturdy wooden spoon to combine.

4. Place a sheet of parchment paper on your work surface and turn the "dough" onto it. Using the parchment to keep your hands clean, press the dough into a 1-inch thick rectangle. Sprinkle the remaining ¼ cup hemp hearts on both sides. Slice into 16 bites.

5. Store in a sealed container in the refrigerator for up to 1 week.

✚
Beauty, Detox, Immune

Sweet and Spicy Curry-Mushroom Nuts

Spicy curry powder can stand up to any mushroom and the intense flavor of molasses, which I love to include in unexpected places for its mineral content. These nuts are delightful as a party snack or chopped and scattered atop a grain bowl or salad for extra crunch.

MAKES: about 3 cups | PREP AND COOK TIME: 30 minutes

1 pound mixed raw nuts

1 tablespoon safflower oil

1 tablespoon yellow curry powder

1 teaspoon blackstrap molasses

1 tablespoon raw or coconut sugar

½ teaspoon sea salt

3 servings powdered mushroom extract

1. Preheat oven to 350°F.

2. Line a baking sheet with parchment paper. Spread the nuts in a single layer and bake for about 10 minutes, until fragrant and lightly browned.

3. Meanwhile, combine the oil, curry, molasses, sugar, and salt in a medium bowl. Toss the nuts in this mixture, then return to the prepared baking sheet. Bake another 10 minutes. Let cool for 10 minutes, then serve immediately, or allow to cool completely and store in sealed container for up to 3 weeks.

✚ Immune

Veggie-Mushroom Flax Crackers

Flaxseed's soluble fiber is the secret to these delicate gluten-free crackers. Packed with vegetables and mushrooms, they're wonderful on their own or spread with Mushroom Hummus (page 149). If you juice regularly, you can swap in veggie pulp for the veggies listed here. Due to the high moisture content of the ingredients, the crackers won't stay crispy for long, but they're so delicious that shouldn't be a problem. Simply dehydrate them again for 30 to 60 minutes if they seem soft. These crackers crumble easily, so spread dips onto them rather than trying to dunk them.

SERVES: 4 | PREP TIME: 15 minutes, plus 4 hours to dehydrate

2 carrots, peeled and chopped

½ medium red or yellow bell pepper, chopped

2 scallions, greens and whites, roughly chopped

1 cup cooked mushrooms or tender mushrooms leftover from cooking broth

½ cup ground flaxseed

2 tablespoons tamari

¼ cup water

1 tablespoon sesame seeds

1. Combine all the ingredients except for the sesame seeds in a food processor. Process until completely smooth.

2. Line a dehydrator sheet with parchment paper. Spread the mixture ¼-inch thick across the parchment using an offset spatula. Sprinkle on the sesame seeds.

3. Dehydrate for 1 hour at 125°F, then score into bite-size pieces. Continue to dehydrate for another 3 hours, until crispy.

4. Let cool, peel off the parchment, and eat immediately or store in an airtight container for up to 5 days.

✚ Immune

Gluten-Free Herbed Mushroom Crackers

These crackers are sturdier than the Veggie-Mushroom Flax Crackers (page 165), so you can dip and dunk to your heart's content. They're also a great way to use up tender mushrooms leftover from making broth. Add dried herbs or spice blends to change up the flavor. The nutritional yeast adds a cheesy taste.

SERVES: 4 | PREP AND COOK TIME: 45 minutes

1 cup almond flour

3 tablespoons olive oil

2 tablespoons ground flaxseed

½ teaspoon salt

¼ cup fresh flat-leaf parsley, minced

2 cloves garlic

¼ cup nutritional yeast (optional)

2 cloves garlic, minced

½ cup cooked mushrooms (such as shiitake, maitake or button), minced or pureed

½ cup water

1. Preheat the oven to 350°F. Line a baking sheet with parchment paper.

2. Combine all the ingredients in a large bowl.

3. Spread the mixture ¼-inch thick across the parchment using an offset spatula. Use a pizza cutter to score the crackers.

4. Bake for about 40 minutes, flipping the crackers over after 20 minutes. Crackers are ready when they are crispy. Let cool, peel off the parchment, and eat immediately or store in an air-tight container for up to five days.

Immune

Shiitake-Avocado Sushi Rolls

I love making sushi rolls at home, especially with these generously seasoned shiitakes. I often use brown rice or quinoa in place of the white rice for more protein and fiber, so feel free to use either of those if desired. Creamy avocado and crunchy scallions are my favorite vegetables in sushi, but add carrots or cucumber if desired.

SERVES: 4 | PREP AND COOK TIME: 30 minutes

1 teaspoon untoasted sesame oil

4 shiitake mushroom caps, thinly sliced

1 clove garlic, minced

½ teaspoon grated fresh ginger

pinch of crushed red pepper

1 teaspoon tamari

4 sheets nori

1 cup cooked sushi rice, prepared according to package directions

4 scallions, trimmed to the width of the nori

1 avocado, sliced into 8 pieces

1. Place a small skillet over medium heat. Heat the oil, then add the shiitakes. Cook, stirring often, for 5 minutes. Stir in the garlic, ginger, crushed red pepper, and tamari, and remove from the heat.

2. Place a sheet of nori flat on a clean, dry cutting board. Spread one quarter of the prepared rice evenly over the nori, leaving a 1-inch strip of the nori bare. Place one quarter of the mushrooms, 1 scallion, and 2 slices of avocado on top of the rice, one inch from the other end of the nori. Roll tightly and evenly, then use a silicone brush to dampen the bare edge of nori. Seal the roll and set aside.

3. Repeat with the remaining rolls. Use a sharp knife to slice into ½-inch pieces.

✚ Cholesterol, Detox, Immune, Skin

Maitake and Spirulina Rice Inari

Inari are fried tofu pockets that have been marinated in a sweet sauce; they're a Japanese snack food or side dish that is often served stuffed with rice and veggies. To offset the sweetness, I rinse my inari, pat them dry, and stuff them with brown rice seasoned with spirulina, sesame, and savory maitake.

SERVES: 4 | PREP AND COOK TIME: 30 minutes

1 cup prepared brown rice

1 teaspoon spirulina

1 teaspoon sesame seeds

1 teaspoon regular sesame oil

½ cup chopped maitake mushrooms

2 teaspoons tamari

8 inari pockets

sriracha, for serving

1. Place the brown rice in a small bowl. Stir in the spirulina and the sesame seeds and set aside.

2. Place a small skillet over medium heat. Heat the oil, then add the maitakes. Cook, stirring often, until they are soft and dark brown, about 5 minutes. Stir in the tamari.

3. Place two tablespoons of rice into each inari pocket, then top with about 1 tablespoon of mushrooms. Drizzle with sriracha if desired.

✚
Blood Sugar, Immune

CHAPTER 8

※

Desserts

Mushrooms are not exactly an ingredient you would expect to find on a dessert menu, and—not to worry—there are no chocolate-dipped portobellos or oyster mushroom pies here. Instead, the recipes use (mostly) mushroom extracts in liquid and powdered form. Many mushrooms are naturally bitter, and they're all somewhat earthy. These recipes are a great way to learn to like those flavors. Keep in mind that the goal of these desserts is not to completely mask the taste of mushrooms, but instead to use their unique flavors to complement other ingredients.

While these recipes are all created using whole foods, avoid giving them a "health halo." They're still treats and should be considered as such, even if each one does contain the natural goodness of mushrooms.

Peanut Butter Chocolate Chip Cookie Dough

Let's just admit it: We all eat raw cookie dough. With this version, there's no need to hide it anymore. There are no raw eggs or flour, both of which can pose health risks when eaten raw; it's just chickpeas and peanut butter powder. Your favorite mushroom powder will blend right in (I've tried chaga, reishi, cordyceps, and turkey tail) to this dessert.

SERVES: 4 to 6 | PREP TIME: 10 minutes

1 (14.5-ounce) can chickpeas, drained and rinsed

¼ cup peanut butter powder

2 tablespoons peanut butter

2 tablespoons coconut sugar or brown sugar

½ teaspoon vanilla extract

3 servings powdered mushroom extract of choice

pinch of sea salt

¼ cup mini chocolate chips

Combine all ingredients except for the chocolate chips in a food processor and process until smooth. Add the chocolate chips, pulse a couple of times to combine, then transfer to a jar or sealed container and refrigerate for up to 5 days.

✚ Immune

CBD Chocolate Coconut Butter

This tastes just like brownie batter, only better! Cannabidiol (CBD) is an active constituent in hemp that has been shown to help conditions like anxiety.[68] From personal experience, I can say I feel calmer and less anxious when I consume CBD. When my friend Andrew started carrying CBD-infused coconut oil at his tea shop, I immediately had to get some. I love combining it with reishi for those times I really need to chill.

SERVES: 1 | PREP TIME: 10 minutes

2 tablespoons coconut butter

1 tablespoon dark cocoa powder

2 teaspoons maple syrup

1 dropper CBD oil

1 serving powdered reishi extract

pinch of sea salt

Combine all the ingredients in a small bowl until smooth. Eat immediately or place on parchment and roll into 1 to 2 balls, then refrigerate until needed.

✚ Adaptogenic, Immune, Mood, Sleep, Stress

Cranberry-Ginger Mushroom Oat Bars

These sweet and spicy ginger bars are one of my favorite afternoon treats. I love the combination of pungent ginger with tart cranberries. The bars are both vegan and gluten-free, with a generous amount of mushroom powder. I like to include a blend of mushrooms in this recipe.

MAKES: 12 to 16 bars | PREP AND COOK TIME: 1 hour

¼ cup coconut oil

⅓ cup maple syrup

⅓ cup coconut sugar or raw sugar

½ cup canned coconut milk

¼ cup apricot jam

¾ teaspoon sea salt

1 teaspoon almond extract

¼ cup water

3 cups old-fashioned oats

6 servings powdered mushroom extract of choice

1 teaspoon baking powder

¼ teaspoon ground ginger

½ cup hemp hearts

½ cup ground flaxseed

½ cup finely chopped crystallized ginger

½ cup dried cranberries

1. Preheat the oven to 325°F. Line a 9 x 13-inch baking pan with parchment paper.

2. Place a medium saucepan over medium heat. Add the coconut oil, maple syrup, sugar, coconut milk, jam, salt, almond extract, and water. Simmer until the sugar dissolves.

3. Grind the oats in a food processor.

4. Transfer the oats to a large bowl along with the mushroom powder, baking powder, ground ginger, hemp, and flaxseed. Pour the maple syrup mixture over the oats. Stir to combine, then fold in the crystallized ginger and cranberries.

5. Spread the oat mixture into the bottom of the prepared baking dish. Top with a piece of parchment, and press down firmly, using a rolling pin or bench scraper if necessary.

6. Bake for about 45 minutes, until golden brown. Let cool completely before slicing or removing from the pan. Store in a sealed container for up to 1 week.

✚
Immune

No-Bake Pumpkin-Chaga Mousse Parfaits

I first whipped up this dessert in pie form for Thanksgiving with friends, but then I decided I don't like oily, buttery graham cracker crusts. To remove the oil needed for a traditional crust, I made these into parfaits, using crumbled graham crackers in place of a crust. Chaga blends well with warm spices, like those traditionally used in pumpkin pie.

SERVES: 4 | PREP AND COOK TIME: 2 hours

⅓ cup melted coconut oil, plus more for the pans

1 teaspoon pumpkin pie spice

1 cup canned pumpkin

¼ cup full-fat coconut milk

1 teaspoon vanilla extract

2 servings powdered chaga extract

¾ cup raw cashews, soaked in hot water for 10 minutes then drained

2 tablespoons lemon juice

¼ cup maple syrup

¼ teaspoon sea salt

4 cinnamon graham crackers, crumbled

ground cinnamon, for garnish

For the caramel:

¼ cup pitted dates, soaked in hot water for at least 10 minutes

¼ teaspoon vanilla extract

½ teaspoon sea salt

1. To prepare the mousse, place the coconut oil a medium saucepan over medium heat. Once melted, add the pumpkin pie spice. Heat until fragrant, about 1 minute, then whisk in the pumpkin, coconut milk, vanilla, and chaga. Cook, stirring often, for about 3 minutes, until the pumpkin is heated through.

2. Transfer to a high-speed blender and add the cashews, lemon juice, maple syrup, and salt. Blend until smooth, pausing as needed to scrape down the sides. Transfer to a bowl, cover, and refrigerate for 2 hours or until ready to serve.

3. To prepare the caramel, in a high-speed blender, puree the dates with ¼ cup of their soaking water, the vanilla, and the salt. Add more water if necessary, and blend until the mixture is smooth and pourable. Transfer to a small bowl.

4. To serve, scoop ⅓ cup of the mousse into each of four parfait dishes or tall glasses. Top each with about one-third of a graham cracker. Repeat with the remaining mousse and graham crackers (you'll have a total of three layers), then drizzle the caramel over the top. Garnish with cinnamon.

✚
Antioxidant, Immune

Reishi-Walnut Chocolates

Long before I knew about the medicinal and healing nature of mushrooms, I knew about the medicinal and healing nature of chocolate. I lean toward more exotic, spicy, and dark varieties, so when I spotted a bar with reishi mushrooms several years ago, I had to try it. The chocolate was rich, dark, and not too sweet, with a lovely texture reminiscent of crispy rice, but finer. I had to create my own version, adding finely chopped walnuts for more texture.

SERVES: 4 to 6 | PREP TIME: 10 minutes, plus 2 hours refrigeration

12 ounces bittersweet chocolate

2 servings powdered reishi extract

¼ cup raw walnuts, finely chopped

2 tablespoons chopped candied ginger (optional)

zest of 1 orange (optional)

sea salt

1. Melt the chocolate in a double boiler or in the microwave. Stir in the reishi and walnuts.

2. Pour into silicone candy molds or a parchment-lined loaf pan. Sprinkle with sea salt.

3. Refrigerate until firm, about 2 hours.

✚ Adaptogenic, Immune, Sleep, Stress

Sexy Truffles

This recipe was among the first I tested, and I shared these truffles with my fellow yoga teachers one afternoon. I didn't have a name for them yet, but after I rattled off the list of ingredients and their potential areas of health support, my friend Melanie bit into one and promptly moaned. "Mmm, sexy truffles," she declared. She's right. These truffles contain the adaptogens maca and cordyceps, which offer up energy (useful if you want to get frisky), along with cayenne to heat things up.

MAKES: 32 | PREP TIME: 10 minutes, plus 1 hour to cool

½ cup full-fat coconut milk

1 tablespoon plus 1 teaspoon maca powder

4 servings powdered cordyceps extract

¼ teaspoon cayenne pepper

12 ounces bittersweet chocolate

¼ cup raw cacao powder or dark cocoa powder

¼ cup hemp hearts

sea salt, to taste

1. Heat the coconut milk over medium-low heat until simmering. Remove from the heat, transfer to a medium bowl, and whisk in the maca, cordyceps, and cayenne, plus a pinch of salt. Stir in the chocolate and add a pinch of salt. Stir until the chocolate is completely melted. Refrigerate for about 1 hour, until slightly firm.

2. Place the cocoa powder, hemp hearts, and a pinch of salt in a shallow dish with a tight-fitting lid. Stir to combine.

3. Scoop 1 tablespoon of the ganache at a time into truffles (I used a small cookie scoop), dropping each one into the cocoa mixture. Working a few at a time, shake gently to coat the truffles. Repeat with the remaining ganache. Cover and refrigerate for up to 4 days.

+ Adaptogenic, Energy, Stress

Spicy Immunity Truffles

February, and thus Valentine's Day, is still solidly in winter, aka cold and flu season. I decided to create a chocolate truffle with plenty of warming, immune-supporting herbs, plus chaga and reishi to spread the love (and hopefully not germs). Subtly sweet and quite decadent, these truffles pack a spicy punch.

MAKES: 32 | PREP TIME: 10 minutes, plus 1 hour to cool

½ cup full-fat coconut milk

3 servings powdered reishi extract

1 serving powdered chaga extract

1 teaspoon ground turmeric

1 teaspoon ground ginger

1 teaspoon ground cinnamon

½ teaspoon ground cloves

pinch of black pepper

12 ounces bittersweet chocolate

¼ cup raw cacao powder or dark cocoa powder

¼ cup hemp hearts

sea salt, to taste

1. Heat the coconut milk over medium-low heat until simmering. Remove from the heat, transfer to a medium bowl, and whisk in the reishi, chaga, turmeric, ginger, cinnamon, cloves, and black pepper, plus a pinch of salt. Stir in the chocolate until it is completely melted. Refrigerate for about 1 hour, until slightly firm.

2. Place the cocoa powder, hemp hearts, and a pinch of salt in a shallow dish with a tight-fitting lid. Stir to combine.

3. Scoop 1 tablespoon of the ganache at a time into truffles (I used a small cookie scoop), dropping each one into the cocoa mixture. Working a few at a time, shake gently to coat the truffles. Repeat with the remaining ganache. Cover and refrigerate for up to 4 days.

✚
Adaptogenic, Antioxidant, Immune

Nerve-Soothing Truffles

Truffles are so easy to make, and mushroom powders blend right in, making them one of my favorite mushroom treats. This version contains calming reishi, lion's mane for the brain and nerves, plus chamomile and lemon balm tinctures—both nervines that can soothe the nerves. Next time you're craving chocolate but feel a little rattled (we all have those days), reach for one of these.

MAKES: 32 | PREP TIME: 10 minutes, plus 1 hour to cool

½ cup full-fat coconut milk

3 servings powdered reishi extract

6 servings powdered lion's mane extract

12 ounces bittersweet chocolate

zest of 1 orange

3 droppers chamomile tincture

3 droppers lemon balm tincture

2 tablespoons dark cocoa powder

2 tablespoons hemp hearts

sea salt, to taste

1. Heat the coconut milk over medium-low heat until simmering. Remove from the heat, transfer to a medium bowl, and whisk in the reishi and lion's mane, plus a pinch of salt. Add the chocolate, orange zest, and chamomile and lemon balm tinctures, and stir until the chocolate is melted. Refrigerate for 1 hour, until slightly firm.

2. Place the cocoa powder, hemp hearts, and a pinch of salt in a shallow dish with a tight-fitting lid. Stir to combine.

3. Scoop 1 tablespoon of the ganache at a time into truffles (I used a small cookie scoop), dropping each one into the cocoa mixture. Working a few at a time, shake gently to coat the truffles. Repeat with the remaining ganache. Cover and refrigerate for up to 4 days.

✚ Adaptogenic, Energy, Memory, Stress

Savasana Truffles

My friend Tish is a born healer—she's not only a yoga teacher, she's also a massage therapist and ayurvedic wellness counselor. So when she asked me to make truffles for her monthly Delicious Yin yoga class, I was honored. I knew exactly which mushroom to use: reishi, of course. After 90 minutes of warm yoga with healing touch, these truffles were a hit. Her students still beg me to sell these truffles.

MAKES: 32 | PREP TIME: 10 minutes, plus 1 hour to cool

½ cup full-fat coconut milk

1 tablespoon powdered reishi extract

12 ounces bittersweet chocolate

¼ cup cacao nibs

¼ cup raw cacao powder or dark cocoa powder

sea salt, to taste

1. Heat the coconut milk over medium-low heat until simmering. Remove from the heat, transfer to a medium bowl, and whisk in the reishi, plus a pinch of salt. Add the chocolate, cacao nibs, and another pinch of salt, then stir until the chocolate is completely melted. Refrigerate for 1 hour, until slightly firm.

2. Place the cocoa powder and a pinch of salt in a shallow dish with a tight-fitting lid. Stir to combine.

3. Scoop 1 tablespoon of the ganache at a time into truffles (I used a small cookie scoop), dropping each one into the cocoa mixture. Working a few at a time, shake gently to coat the truffles. Repeat with the remaining ganache. Cover and refrigerate for up to 4 days.

✚ Adaptogenic, Immune, Nervous System, Sleep

Gingerbread Meltaways

Gingerbread's signature intensity comes from a combination of tinny, strongly flavored blackstrap molasses and warm, immune-boosting herbs and spices. Molasses is rare among sweeteners in that it is rich in minerals like calcium, iron, and potassium. Feel free to adjust the spices in these meltaways to match your favorite gingerbread recipe; it seems every family has their own special spice blend. I added a generous amount of reishi and turkey tail to these meltaways to further support the immune system.

MAKES: 16 | PREP TIME: 10 minutes, plus 1 hour to chill

½ cup raw nut butter

½ cup unrefined coconut oil, melted

2 tablespoons maple syrup

3 servings powdered reishi extract

3 servings powdered turkey tail extract

2 tablespoons blackstrap molasses

½ teaspoon ground turmeric

1 tablespoon ground cinnamon

1 tablespoon ground ginger

1 tablespoon ground allspice

1 teaspoon ground nutmeg

1 teaspoon ground cloves

pinch of black pepper

hemp hearts, for sprinkling

sea salt, for sprinkling

1. Whisk the nut butter and coconut oil together in a medium bowl, then add the rest of the ingredients, except for the hemp hearts and sea salt.

2. Place a silicone candy mold on a tray or baking sheet. Use a tablespoon to pour the mixture into the molds, leaving space at the top of each one. Sprinkle with the hemp hearts and a pinch of sea salt.

3. Freeze or refrigerate until firm, at least 1 hour.

4. Remove from molds and transfer to a sealed container. Freeze or refrigerate for up to 1 month. They melt slightly at room temperature due to the coconut oil.

✚ Adaptogenic, Bones and Joints, Immune

Memory Meltaways

Lion's mane and reishi are the stars of these tasty memory-supporting meltaways, made with nut butter and coconut oil. I also include holy basil for stress support (since stress can impact memory) or gotu kola, which aids circulation in the brain. I regularly make these meltaways with several combinations of herbs and mushrooms based on my mood and health. The mushroom powders are easy to mix in, making these a great treat for those who are new to mushrooms.

MAKES: 16 | PREP TIME: 10 minutes, plus 1 hour to chill

½ cup raw nut butter

½ cup unrefined coconut oil, melted

2 tablespoons maple syrup

3 servings powdered lion's mane extract

1 teaspoon powdered reishi extract

4 droppers holy basil or gotu kola tincture

hemp hearts, for sprinkling

sea salt, for sprinkling

1. Whisk the nut butter and coconut oil together in a medium bowl, then add the rest of the ingredients, except for the hemp hearts and sea salt.

2. Place a silicone candy mold on a tray or baking sheet. Use a tablespoon to pour the mixture into the molds, leaving space at the top of each one. Sprinkle with the hemp hearts and a pinch of sea salt.

3. Freeze or refrigerate until firm, at least 1 hour.

4. Remove from molds and transfer to a sealed container. Freeze or refrigerate for up to 1 month. They melt slightly at room temperature due to the coconut oil.

✚ Adaptogenic, Immune, Memory, Stress

Recovery Meltaways

These "fat bombs" are a snack staple for those following a ketogenic diet. While I am definitely not keto, I love that each bite is rich and satisfying. I keep a batch in the fridge and grab one when I need something to tide me over until mealtime. Here, I added anti-inflammatory herbs, spices, and mushrooms to help aid recovery after a tough workout.

MAKES: 16 | PREP TIME: 10 minutes, plus 1 hour to chill

½ cup raw nut butter

½ cup unrefined coconut oil, melted

2 tablespoons maple syrup

1 tablespoon ground turmeric

1 tablespoon ground ginger

1 tablespoon beet powder

3 servings powdered chaga extract

3 servings powdered cordyceps extract

pinch of sea salt

1. Whisk the nut butter and coconut oil together in a small bowl, then add the rest of the ingredients.

2. Place a silicone candy mold on a tray or baking sheet. Pour the mixture into the molds, leaving space at the top of each one. Freeze or refrigerate until firm, at least one hour.

3. Remove from the molds and transfer to a sealed container. Freeze or refrigerate for up to 1 month. They melt slightly at room temperature due to the coconut oil.

+
Antioxidant, Energy, Immune, Stress

Brain-Boosting Macaroons

Given that lion's mane mushrooms look so similar to a coconut macaroon, I knew I had to make macaroons with my favorite brain booster. Gluten-free and vegan, these cookies use maple syrup in place of sugar, with a generous amount of both lion's mane and cordyceps powders. I also offer MCT (medium-chain triglyceride) oil as a substitute for coconut oil, as some say it can give the brain a boost (though no studies have yet proven that).

MAKES: 16 | PREP TIME: 10 minutes, plus 1 hour to chill

1 ½ cups almond meal

1 cup unsweetened shredded coconut

¼ teaspoon salt

4 servings powdered lion's mane extract

2 servings powdered cordyceps extract

½ cup maple syrup

1 teaspoon vanilla or almond extract

2 tablespoons melted coconut oil or MCT oil

1. Combine the almond meal, coconut, salt, and lion's mane and cordyceps extracts in a medium bowl. Combine the maple syrup, vanilla or almond extract, and coconut or MCT oil in a small bowl. Fold the wet ingredients into the dry until combined, then use an ice-cream or cookie scoop to form macaroon-shaped cookies. Place on a Teflex-lined dehydrator tray.

2. Dehydrate at 120°F for 4 to 6 hours, until they reach the desired texture. If you don't have a dehydrator, bake at 150°F for 2 to 3 hours. Keep refrigerated in an airtight container for up to 1 week.

✚ Adaptogenic, Energy, Immune, Memory, Stress

Adaptogenic Chia Pudding

Chia pudding is a trendy treat, and for good reason. It's thick and creamy, with plenty of fiber, protein, and omega-3 fatty acids. This version contains three adaptogens—reishi, cordyceps, and ashwagandha—plus dark cocoa powder, making it perfect for days when you can feel your stress level rising.

SERVES: 4 | PREP TIME: 10 minutes, plus 1 hour to chill

½ cup chia seeds

½ teaspoon vanilla extract (optional)

2 tablespoons maple syrup or 2 pitted dates soaked and blended with water

1 tablespoon dark cocoa powder

1⅔ cups milk

1 teaspoon ashwagandha powder

1 teaspoon powdered reishi extract

1 serving powdered cordyceps extract

pinch of salt

For garnish:

dark chocolate shavings

candied ginger or orange zest

chopped pistachios

1. Combine all the ingredients in a medium bowl, then stir every couple of minutes for about 10 minutes. Cover and refrigerate for at least an hour, or overnight.

2. If the pudding is too thick, whisk in a couple of tablespoons of water or milk before serving. Garnish as desired and eat immediately, or refrigerate for up to 3 days.

✚ Adaptogenic, Energy, Immune, Mood, Stress

Panic-Button Cashew Butter Cups

If you're someone who reaches for chocolate when the world asks too much of you, this is a treat for you. Cashews are a good source of magnesium, which is known as the relaxation mineral for its role in nerve function. I added reishi and ashwagandha to boost the chill, plus cordyceps for energy.

MAKES: 16 | PREP TIME: 10 minutes, plus 1 hour, 10 minutes to chill

12 ounces bittersweet chocolate

½ cup unrefined coconut oil, melted, divided

½ cup cashew butter

2 tablespoons maple syrup

1 serving powdered cordyceps extract

3 servings powdered reishi extract

1 teaspoon powdered ashwagandha root

pinch of sea salt

1. Microwave the chocolate with 1 teaspoon of the coconut oil. Start with 30 seconds, then stir and heat for another 15 seconds at a time, until the chocolate is about two-thirds of the way melted. The residual heat will melt the chocolate the rest of the way.

2. Whisk the nut butter and remaining coconut oil together in a small bowl, then stir in the rest of the ingredients.

3. Place a silicone candy mold on a tray or baking sheet, or line a mini muffin tin with paper liners. Place about 1 tablespoon chocolate into the bottom of each liner or compartment, making sure you smooth it to the edges. Freeze for 10 minutes.

4. Top each compartment with about 2 teaspoons of the nut butter mixture, then another tablespoon of chocolate.

5. Freeze or refrigerate until firm, at least 1 hour.

6. Remove the cashew butter cups from molds and transfer to a sealed container. Freeze or refrigerate for up to 1 month.

+ Adaptogenic, Energy, Immune, Stress

Reishi Almond "Snickers" Bites

Now these really satisfy! These bites take 15 minutes to prepare—max—and they're the perfect two-bite treats when you want just a little something sweet. Dates taste so close to caramel, with far less effort required. The bitterness of reishi balances well with the rest of the ingredients.

MAKES: 24 | PREP TIME: 15 minutes, plus 1 hour to chill

12 pitted dates

48 almonds

1 ½ cups bittersweet chocolate chips

3 servings powdered reishi extract

1 tablespoon coconut oil

sea salt, for sprinkling

1. Line a baking sheet with parchment paper. Split the dates in half, and place them on the prepared baking sheet in a single layer, pit side up.

2. Place two almonds in each date half.

3. Place the chocolate chips in a small, microwave-safe bowl. Heat in 10-second increments, stirring each time, until mostly melted, then stir in the reishi and coconut oil, along with a pinch of salt.

4. Spoon 1 tablespoon of the melted chocolate over the top of each date. Top with a sprinkle of sea salt, if desired.

5. Let cool, then eat immediately or cover and refrigerate for up to 3 days.

✚ Adaptogenic, Immune, Mood, Sleep, Stress

Joyful Almond-Coconut Bites

These "joyful" almond bites are perfectly sweet with no refined sugar (aside from what might be in your chocolate). Toasting the coconut and adding almond extract gives these a more complex flavor beyond simply being "sweet." I used a simple round candy mold to make these bites.

MAKES: 16 | PREP TIME: 20 minutes, plus time to chill

1 cup unsweetened coconut chips or large flakes

¾ cup dates, pitted and soaked in ¾ cup hot water for at least 20 minutes

4 servings powdered reishi or chaga extract

½ cup bittersweet chocolate chips

1 teaspoon coconut oil

1 teaspoon almond extract

pinch of sea salt

16 roasted unsalted almonds

1. Place a small skillet over medium heat. Add the coconut and cook for 5 to 7 minutes, shaking often, until it is fragrant and toasted.

2. Meanwhile, drain the dates well and transfer to the bowl of a food processor. Pulse until roughly chopped, add the reishi or chaga, and pulse again until the mixture forms a ball that's uniform in texture.

3. Melt the chocolate with the coconut oil, using the microwave or a small saucepan set over low heat. Once melted, add the salt and remove from the heat.

4. Once the coconut is toasted, add it to the food processor along with the almond extract and another pinch of salt. Pulse until thoroughly combined with the dates but not pureed. The coconut should still have some texture.

5. Scoop about 2 tablespoons of the date and coconut mixture into your hands. Roll into a ball, then slightly flatten it so it can fit comfortably inside a silicone candy mold. Place on a sheet of parchment. Repeat with the remaining date and coconut mixture. Press an almond on top of each bite.

6. Fill 16 cups of a candy mold with 1 teaspoon each of the melted chocolate. Place one ball into each prepared cup, then drizzle each with ½ teaspoon of melted chocolate. Let cool completely, remove from the candy molds, and store in a sealed container in the fridge for up to 1 week.

✚
Immune

Tahini-Chocolate No-Bake Cookies

I have fond memories of making no-bake cookies with my mom when I was a kid. It wasn't until the first time I tried to make them on my way that I realized my mom cut way back on the sugar, but I prefer them her way. Here, they still contain less sugar but get an upgrade, thanks to tahini in place of peanut butter and a trio of mushroom powders. I prefer almond extract as I think it adds more flavor, but you can use vanilla instead.

MAKES: 16 | PREP TIME: 10 minutes, plus 1 hour to chill

½ cup coconut sugar

¼ cup coconut milk

2 tablespoons coconut oil

1¼ cups old-fashioned oats

¼ cup almond meal

3 tablespoons dark cocoa powder

½ serving powdered maitake extract

1 serving powdered turkey tail extract

½ serving powdered cordyceps extract

½ cup tahini

1 teaspoon vanilla or almond extract

pinch of sea salt

1. Line a baking sheet with parchment paper.

2. Combine the coconut sugar, coconut milk, and coconut oil in a medium saucepan over medium heat. Cook, stirring constantly, until it reaches a boil, then let boil for 1 minute.

3. Remove from the heat and stir in remaining ingredients. Drop tablespoons of the mixture onto the prepared baking sheet and let harden at room temperature. Refrigerate for up to 3 days in a sealed container.

✚ Adaptogenic, Cardiovascular, Energy, Immune

Chilled-Out Avocado Chocolate Mousse

Chocolate releases feel-good hormones, and it also has been shown to lower inflammation associated with heart disease.[69] Here, the usual cream in chocolate mousse is swapped for heart-healthy avocado, which also adds fiber. CBD oil, reishi, and lion's mane increase the feel-good and chill-out factor of this simple dessert.

SERVES: 1 or 2 | PREP TIME: 10 minutes, plus optional 1 hour to chill

1 avocado, pitted and peeled

1 tablespoon maple syrup, or more to taste

2 tablespoons dark cocoa powder or raw cacao powder

1 serving powdered lion's mane extract

1 serving powdered reishi extract

1 dropper CBD oil

¼ cup unsweetened almond milk

pinch of sea salt

hemp hearts, for garnish

flaked sea salt, for garnish

Combine all the ingredients except the garnishes in a food processor or blender and process until smooth. Transfer to two bowls, and refrigerate for up to 12 hours or eat immediately, garnished with hemp hearts and flaked sea salt.

✚ Adaptogenic, Energy, Immune, Memory, Mood, Stress

Mushroom Chocolate Cheesecake

This raw vegan cheesecake is decadent and packed with real food ingredients. It gets an immune and mood boost from reishi and chaga, but you can swap in another mushroom powder if desired.

SERVES: 4 | PREP TIME: 30 minutes, plus 1 hour to freeze

For the crust:

½ cup pitted dates, soaked in hot water for 10 minutes then drained

1 cup raw walnuts

2 servings powdered chaga extract

2 tablespoons dark cocoa powder or raw cacao powder

⅛ teaspoon sea salt

For the filling:

5 tablespoons melted coconut oil, plus more for the pans

¾ cup raw cashews, soaked in hot water for 10 minutes then drained

2 tablespoons lemon juice

¼ cup maple syrup

2 servings powdered reishi extract

¼ cup dark cocoa powder or raw cacao powder

¼ cup full-fat coconut milk

2 tablespoons cacao nibs, for topping

1. To prepare the crust, pulse the dates and walnuts together in a food processor until roughly chopped. Add the remaining ingredients and pulse until finely chopped and thoroughly combined.

2. Grease a 9-inch pie pan with coconut oil, then press the crust mixture evenly into the bottom and sides of the pan. It should be about ¼-inch thick. Freeze while you prep the filling.

3. To prepare the filling, blend all the ingredients except the cacao nibs together until smooth, pausing as needed to scrape down the sides.

4. Once the filling is completely smooth, remove the crust from the freezer. Pour the filling into the prepared crust, then sprinkle on the cacao nibs.

5. Freeze for 1 hour before serving. If not serving immediately, refrigerate until ready to eat. Cover and refrigerate for up to 4 days or freeze
   for up to three months.

✚
Adaptogenic, Antioxidant, Immune, Sleep, Stress

Chocolate Magic Mushroom Shell

Let's be clear: There are no "magic" mushrooms in this recipe. It's a mushroom-infused version of magic shell chocolate crackle to pour over ice cream and other frozen treats. I love it with a combo of chaga and reishi atop banana "nice" cream (pureed frozen banana). Use bittersweet chocolate to highlight the flavor of the mushrooms and offer a nice contrast to your sweet frozen dessert.

MAKES: ½ cup | PREP TIME: 5 minutes

2 tablespoons coconut oil

½ cup bittersweet chocolate chips

1 serving powdered reishi extract

1 serving powdered chaga extract

pinch of sea salt

1. In a small microwave-safe bowl, melt the coconut oil in the microwave. Stir in the chocolate chips, microwaving in 15-second increments and stirring between each increment, until the chocolate is two-thirds melted, 30 to 45 seconds. The residual heat will finish melting the chocolate. Whisk in the reishi and chaga extracts and salt.

2. Let cool slightly and drizzle over ice cream or frozen treats immediately. Cover and refrigerate any leftovers for up to 1 week, re-melting as needed.

✚ Adaptogenic, Immune

Adaptogenic Mushroom Fudge

This simple fudge satisfies a sweet tooth with real food. The combo of nut butter and coconut oil provide satiating fat and a whole lot of stress-busting adaptogens. Cordyceps and maca give you a nice energy boost too.

SERVES: 4 to 6 | PREP TIME: 10 minutes, plus 1 hour to chill

½ cup raw nut butter

½ cup unrefined coconut oil, melted

⅓ cup raw cacao powder

2 tablespoons maple syrup

2 tablespoons maca

1 serving powdered turkey tail extract

1 serving powdered shiitake extract

1 serving powdered cordyceps extract

For garnish:

flaked sea salt

cacao nibs

ground cinnamon

cayenne pepper

ground ginger

1. Whisk the nut butter and coconut oil together in a small bowl, then add the rest of the ingredients. Place a silicone candy mold on a tray or baking sheet.

2. Pour the mixture into the molds, leaving space at the top of each one. Garnish as desired.

3. Freeze or refrigerate until firm, then remove from the molds. Freeze or refrigerate for up to 1 month in a sealed container. They melt slightly at room temperature due to the coconut oil.

✚ Adaptogenic, Cholesterol, Detox, Energy, Immune, Stress

Laquiregme Mushroom Butter

CHAPTER 9

Condiments, Flavorings, and Other Infusions

With a little bit of time and little bit more patience, you can elevate the flavor of pantry—and liquor cabinet—staples simply by adding mushrooms. This chapter is not about instant gratification. These recipes are projects that may take weeks to yield a finished product (but thankfully not much hands-on work).

If you're trying to introduce skeptics to the wonder of mushrooms, start here. Give a bottle of mushroom-infused vodka as a hostess gift, share a jar of stock powder with a coworker, or finish any savory dish with a pat of mushroom butter.

Chanterelle or Shiitake Vodka

Herbal tinctures are basically just infused vodka or grain alcohol used for a medicinal purpose. However, this recipe is intended more for culinary (or mixology) purposes than purely medicinal ones. There's a recipe for making mushroom tinctures on page 206, and while this vodka does deliver plenty of mushroom flavor, I prefer to use it in cocktails than as a supplement.

MAKES: 1 cup | PREP TIME: 5 minutes, plus 2 weeks to steep

1 cup organic vodka

1 ounce dried chanterelles or shiitakes, roughly chopped

1. Pour the vodka into a pint jar, then add the mushrooms.

2. Cover, shake to combine, and let sit in a cool, dark place for up to 2 weeks. Strain, reserving the mushrooms for another dish if desired. Store for up to 1 year.

✚ Cardiovascular, Detox, Immune

Mushroom-Infused Sherry

You've noticed by now that I love to cook mushrooms with sherry. This simple recipe infuses dry sherry with mushrooms to add flavor and their alcohol-soluble components to any dish. It makes a lovely gift, but be sure to allow plenty of time for it to steep.

MAKES: 1 (375-ml) bottle | PREP TIME: 5 minutes, plus 2 weeks to steep

1 (375-ml) bottle dry sherry

1 cup dried mushrooms, any variety, roughly chopped

1. Pour the sherry into a large jar, then add the mushrooms.

2. Cover, shake to combine, and let sit in a cool, dark place for up to 2 weeks. Strain, reserving the mushrooms for another dish if desired. Store for up to 1 year.

✚
Immune

Mushroom Stock Powder

This recipe yields powdered mushrooms, which shouldn't be confused with powdered mushroom extracts. This powder is meant to be mixed with boiling water or added to soups and stews for extra mushroom flavor when you haven't had time to make stock. The nutritional yeast adds extra umami; there's not enough in this recipe to yield many nutritional benefits.

MAKES: 1 cup | PREP TIME: 5 minutes

½ pound dried mushrooms

¼ cup nutritional yeast

1 tablespoon salt

1 teaspoon onion powder

½ teaspoon garlic powder

1 teaspoon black pepper

1 teaspoon dried thyme

1 teaspoon dried rosemary

2 bay leaves

1. Grind all ingredients in a clean coffee grinder or blender. Transfer to jar and store for up to 1 year.

2. To use, add 1 teaspoon powder to 1 cup boiling water.

✚
Immune

Mushroom Butter

I have to give full credit to my husband, Sam, for this recipe. I made garlic bread one night, after which he suggested I make mushroom butter. It was a simple, brilliant idea, and this recipe is now a staple in our home. (We use homemade "butter" made from coconut and olive oils.)

MAKES: ½ pound | PREP AND COOK TIME: 20 minutes, plus time to chill

1 tablespoon safflower oil

2 cups tender mushrooms, minced in a food processor

1 tablespoon dried mushrooms, coarsely ground and soaked in 2 tablespoons of water for at least 10 minutes

1 tablespoon fresh rosemary, minced

⅛ teaspoon pepper

2 tablespoons dry sherry

1 garlic clove, minced

1 cup (2 sticks) unsalted butter, at room temperature

salt, to taste

1. Place a medium skillet over medium heat. Add the oil, then the fresh and dried mushrooms and rosemary. Add a pinch of salt and the pepper.

2. Cook, stirring occasionally, for about 10 minutes, until the mushrooms have softened and released most of their liquid.

3. Add the sherry, scraping the bottom of the pan to remove any brown bits. Cook about 5 minutes more, until the mixture is quite dry.

4. Stir in the garlic, cook for 1 minute, then remove from heat.

5. Transfer to a food processor, along with the butter. Pulse to combine, and salt to taste.

6. Once thoroughly combined, transfer to a sheet of parchment, roll into a log, and refrigerate until firm.

7. Refrigerate for up to 1 week or freeze for up to 3 months.

✚ Immune

Life Happens Syrup

In my life, this syrup is more medicinal than culinary. I keep a bottle in my fridge for rough days when I need a little pick-me-up. Add a spoonful to tea or yogurt, or take it straight up. It helps me adapt and balance when life happens (or should I say when shiitake happens?). Passionflower is my "spirit herb" for mood and anxiety, and chamomile is a runner-up. Along with lemon balm, chamomile helps ease a nervous tummy. I added eleuthero, which is known as Siberian ginseng, to support my body during times of stress.

MAKES: ½ cup | PREP TIME: 5 minutes

¼ cup honey or maple syrup

4 droppers reishi liquid extract

4 droppers eleuthero tincture

4 droppers passionflower tincture

2 droppers chamomile tincture

2 droppers lemon balm tincture

Shake all ingredients together in a small bottle. Keep refrigerated for up to 3 months.

✚
Energy, Immune, Sleep, Stress

Mushroom Soy Sauce

This sauce is so simple yet adds a deep, rich mushroom flavor to even the humblest of dishes. I like to drizzle it over plain grilled tofu, steamed greens, and brown rice, along with good toasted sesame oil. If you prefer, you can make this recipe with liquid aminos, either Bragg's or coconut.

MAKES: 1 cup | PREP TIME: 1 hour, plus 2 weeks to steep

1 cup dried mushrooms, such as maitake or shiitake, sliced or coarsely ground

2 cups water

2 cups soy sauce

1. In a small pan, simmer the mushrooms in 2 cups of water for 30 minutes.

2. Bring to a boil, reduce to a simmer, and cook until the liquid reduces to 1 cup. Add the soy sauce and let simmer for 2 minutes.

3. Pour into a canning jar.

4. Let cool, then cover and let sit in a cool, dark place for 2 weeks or up to 1 month.

5. Strain, reserving the mushrooms. (They can be frozen and added to future soups, stock bases, etc.) Transfer to a bottle and refrigerate for up to 6 months.

✚
Immune

Porcini Tapenade

Though you could use any tender mushroom in this tapenade, I find porcini to be my favorite. They are so flavorful (and underappreciated in the States), and they add an unrivaled intensity. If you find them fresh, you're in luck—but simply sauté those. For this recipe, opt for frozen, which are available at Trader Joe's. You can swap in another mushroom if need be. I love to serve this in endive leaves with a dollop of cashew cheese.

MAKES: 1 cup | PREP AND COOK TIME: 20 minutes

2 tablespoons olive oil

½ cup frozen chopped porcini mushrooms

1 teaspoon dried oregano

3 cloves garlic, minced

½ cup pitted kalamata olives

1 tablespoon lemon juice

⅛ teaspoon black pepper

6 basil leaves

2 tablespoons flat-leaf parsley leaves

1. Place a small skillet over medium heat. Add the oil, mushrooms, and oregano. Cook, stirring often, for about 10 minutes, until the mushrooms are cooked through and starting to get some color.

2. Transfer the mixture, including any liquid, to a food processor. Pulse a few times, then add the remaining ingredients. Pulse again, then process until combined but not smooth.

3. Serve immediately, or refrigerate for up to 5 days.

✚
Cardiovascular, Immune

Dairy-Free Cream-of-Mushroom Soup Base

I am not ashamed to say I cooked with condensed cream of mushroom soup for much of my life. When I gave up dairy, I needed a substitute, so I developed this recipe to add creaminess to casseroles, dips, and the like. It's not meant to be the best mushroom soup of your life. Each portion is meant to replace one can of condensed soup in a recipe.

MAKES: 4 portions | PREP AND COOK TIME: 30 minutes

1 tablespoon olive oil

1 large onion, chopped

3 cloves garlic, minced

2 tablespoons chopped fresh herbs (any combination of sage, thyme, rosemary, and parsley)

½ teaspoon black pepper

4 cups sliced mushrooms (cremini, shiitake, maitake, etc.)

1 (14.5-ounce) can white beans, drained and rinsed

¼ cup cashews, soaked in hot water for 30 minutes and drained

1 cup mushroom broth

1 tablespoon tamari

2 tablespoons nutritional yeast

1. Place a large pot over medium-high heat. Add the oil, then the onions. Cook, stirring often, for about 8 minutes, until the onions are soft. Add the garlic, lower the heat to medium, then cook another 2 minutes, until fragrant.

2. Add the herbs, pepper, and mushrooms. Stir well, and cook for about 10 minutes, continuing to stir occasionally, until the mushrooms are dark brown and soft.

3. While the mushrooms are cooking, blend the beans and cashews with the broth in a blender or food processor. Blend until completely smooth and thick (barely pourable).

4. Remove the mushroom mixture from heat and add half to the bean mixture, along with the tamari and nutritional yeast. Pulse several times until combined. Transfer to the pot, and fold into the remaining mushrooms. Season to taste with salt and pepper.

5. Let cool, and divide into ½-cup portions. Use in any recipe that might call for condensed cream of mushroom soup. Refrigerate for up to 3 days or freeze for up to 3 months.

✚
Immune

Basic Reishi or Chaga Extract (Dual Extraction)

To get the most from your reishi and chaga mushrooms, opt for a dual extraction using alcohol and water. This two-step process helps ensure you get the alcohol- and water-soluble parts of the mushroom. This recipe uses the simplest method, which is deliberately vague so you can scale it up or down. It can be used in recipes or as medicine.

Throughout my research, I kept reading that vitamin C increases absorption of mushroom extracts, so I often dilute mine with a bit of orange or lime juice.

MAKES: servings vary | PREP AND COOK TIME: 1 hour, plus 1 month to steep

dried chaga or reishi mushrooms

organic vodka

2 quarts water

1. Fill a canning jar halfway with mushrooms.

2. Fill the rest of the jar with vodka, leaving ½ inch of space at the top.

3. Allow to steep for 1 month in a cool, dark place. Give it a shake every day or so.

4. After a month, strain the mushrooms. Reserve the vodka infusion.

5. Bring the water to a boil in a large pot, then add the mushrooms strained from the vodka. Let simmer until the water reduces by half to three-quarters, leaving no more than 2 cups. Add water as needed if necessary.

6. Let the water cool, strain and discard the mushrooms, and combine the water extract with the infused vodka. The mixture needs to be at least 25 percent to be safely stored at room temperature.

✚ CHAGA: Immune, Antioxidant; REISHI: Immune, Sleep, Stress, Adaptogenic

CHAPTER 10

Broths

Broths are a traditional way to consume mushrooms, especially while convalescing. This chapter is as healing and medicinal as it is culinary. Slowly simmering mushrooms allows the nutrients more time to be released, and broths are generally easy to digest. Most of the broths use only mushrooms, but Abby Artemisia shared recipes for her two favorite seasonal bone broths with mushrooms too.

Spring Bone Broth with Mushrooms

Abby Artemisia created two seasonal bone broths using mushrooms; this one uses a variety of great tonifying herbs, especially good for spring. (For her Cold and Flu Season Mushroom Bone Broth, see page 213.) Abby starts taking nettles about a month before allergy season starts, to prevent hay fever and keep her sinuses healthy. She included burdock to help with spring allergies too. Burdock supports the liver to process everything coming into the body in an efficient healthy way, instead of attacking unnecessarily, leading to allergy symptoms. Since spring is the tail end of cold and flu season, she also included kombu and astragalus, which she says is "one of the most tonifying Chinese food herbs I know."

Here are her time-tested tips for making bone broth: "Over the years, I've found it's easiest and most economical to make this by buying whole chickens, cooking and eating them, and saving the bones in a bag in the freezer. I save my compostable scraps too, like kale, chard, and broccoli stalks, carrot tops, and onion, garlic, and squash skins. Those go in a separate bag in the freezer. When I'm ready to make broth, I'll pull both bags out and let them thaw."

MAKES: servings vary | PREP AND COOK TIME: 10 minutes, plus 8 to 24 hours to cook

bones of 1 small chicken

1 tablespoon apple cider vinegar

3 cups vegetable scraps

1 stalk fresh celery, coarsely chopped

2 carrots, coarsely chopped

1 medium onion, chopped

4 cloves garlic, chopped

¼ cup dried chaga mushroom granules

½ cup dried lion's mane mushrooms

½ cup dried maitake mushrooms

6 (1-inch) slices reishi mushrooms

1 cup fresh stinging nettle leaves

1 tablespoon sliced burdock root

¼ cup dried astragalus root

10 black peppercorns

1-inch piece kombu seaweed

1 gallon filtered water

salt, to taste

1. Smash the chicken bones with a meat mallet to release the marrow.

2. Add the bones and all the other ingredients into a large stock pot or crock pot along with 1 gallon of filtered water. Let it sit for an hour

to allow the vinegar to start extracting the minerals. Cook at a low simmer for 8 to 24 hours.

3. Strain, season to taste with salt, and pour the broth into jars. Cover and refrigerate for up to 1 week or freeze for up to 3 months.

✚
Immune

Spring Mushroom Broth

This broth contains my favorite spring herbs—tarragon, dill, thyme, and parsley—plus fresh, green veggies like fennel, leek, and celery. Fennel supports digestion and adds a light licorice flavor, while celery and leeks are naturally detoxifying. This is a place to use your workhorse mushrooms—shiitake, maitake, and cremini—and save the tender wild ones that pop up in spring for more delicate, quicker-cooking dishes. I tend not to add the tough, immune-boosting mushrooms to my spring broth, but that's always an option.

MAKES: servings vary | PREP AND COOK TIME: 10 minutes, plus 4 to 24 hours to cook

1 pound mixed mushrooms, including shiitake, maitake, and cremini, roughly chopped

3 sprigs fresh tarragon

2 sprigs fresh dill

3 sprigs fresh thyme

4 sprigs fresh flat-leaf parsley

6 cloves garlic, smashed

1 leek, whites and light green parts, roughly chopped

1 fennel bulb with stalks, roughly chopped

2 stalks celery with leaves, roughly chopped

salt and pepper, to taste

1. Place all the ingredients in slow cooker or large stock pot. Cover with water and bring to a simmer. Simmer for at least four hours on low heat, but preferably overnight.

2. Season to taste with salt and pepper.

3. Let cool, strain the broth, and pour into quart-size canning jars, leaving ½ inch of headspace at the top of each. Refrigerate for up to 5 days or freeze for up to 3 months.

✚ Digestion, Immune

Summer Harvest Mushroom Broth

We tend not to crave warm broths in summer—or think much about immune health on sunny days—but I try to make this summer harvest broth a couple of times a month. I use it to create light vegetable soups, to thin out pasta sauces, or simply for sipping, warm or chilled. It has a subtle tomato flavor, as well as the flavor of Italian herbs. Since this broth contains only tender mushrooms, I don't usually cook it longer than four hours, but you can if desired.

MAKES: servings vary | PREP AND COOK TIME: 4 hours, 10 minutes

1 pound mixed mushrooms, including shiitake, maitake, and cremini, roughly chopped

3 sprigs fresh thyme

1 tablespoon fresh oregano

4 sprigs fresh flat-leaf parsley

6 cloves garlic, smashed

1 large yellow onion, peeled and quartered

2 stalks celery with leaves, roughly chopped

2 plum tomatoes, roughly chopped

4 sprigs fresh basil

salt and pepper, to taste

1. Place all the ingredients in slow cooker or large stock pot. Cover with water and bring to a simmer. Simmer for at least four hours on low heat. Season to taste with salt and pepper.

2. Let cool, strain, and pour into quart-size canning jars, leaving ½ inch of headspace at the top of each. Refrigerate for up to 5 days or freeze for up to 3 months.

✚ Immune

Fall and Winter Mushroom Broth

Fall and winter are the seasons when I crave broth daily. I fortify mine with tough and tender mushrooms, plus loads of aromatic herbs and vegetables. I include ginger and turmeric because they're a powerful duo for antioxidant and anti-inflammatory support, plus my favorite immunoprotective herb, astragalus.

MAKES: servings vary | PREP AND COOK TIME: 10 minutes, plus 4 to 24 hours to cook

1 pound mixed mushrooms, including shiitake, maitake, and cremini, roughly chopped

1-inch cube or 2 slices dried reishi mushrooms

2 or 3 dried turkey tail mushrooms

6 sprigs fresh rosemary

¼ cup fresh sage leaves, chopped

2 tablespoons fresh marjoram leaves

6 sprigs fresh thyme

8 sprigs fresh flat-leaf parsley

6 cloves garlic, smashed

4 astragalus slices

2-inch piece fresh ginger, roughly chopped

1 tablespoon ground turmeric

1 large yellow onion, peeled and quartered

10 black peppercorns

3 bay leaves

1. Place all the ingredients in slow cooker or large stock pot. Cover with water and bring to a simmer. Simmer for at least four hours on low heat, but preferably overnight. Season to taste with salt and pepper.

2. Let cool, strain, and pour into quart-size canning jars, leaving ½ inch of headspace at the top of each. Refrigerate for up to 5 days or freeze for up to 3 months or freeze for up to 3 months.

✚ Adaptogenic, Immune

Cold and Flu Season Mushroom Bone Broth

This is Abby Artemisia's go-to bone broth during the colder months: "The herbs in this soup are designed to help you batten down the hatches for the upcoming cold and flu season. The garlic, turmeric, and ginger all have differing degrees of antibacterial, antiviral, and antibiotic activity and are superboosters for the immune system. They are also awesome at increasing circulation and warmth in the body, a great thing to have for the upcoming drop in temperatures. The black pepper helps your body better absorb the turmeric and ginger and also adds some nice heat. Though all these herbs are warming, none of them are too spicy. However, you can add some cayenne or your hot pepper of choice if you like it hot!"

MAKES: servings vary | PREP AND COOK TIME: 10 minutes, plus 8 to 24 hours to cook

bones from 1 small chicken

1 tablespoon apple cider vinegar

2 stalks fresh celery, coarsely chopped

3 carrots, coarsely chopped

1 medium onion, unpeeled and chopped coarsely

1 head garlic, unpeeled and chopped coarsely

¼ cup chaga mushroom granules

10 medium dried shiitake mushrooms, broken into chunks

3 tablespoons dried turmeric or 5 inches fresh turmeric root, coarsely chopped

3 tablespoons dried ginger or 5 inches fresh ginger root, coarsely chopped

6 (1-inch) slices reishi mushrooms

15 black peppercorns

1 piece kombu seaweed

1 gallon filtered water

salt, to taste

1. Smash the chicken bones with a meat mallet to release the marrow.

2. Add the bones and all the other ingredients into a large stock pot or slow cooker. Let it sit for an hour to allow the vinegar to start extracting the minerals. Cook at a low simmer for 8 to 24 hours.

3. Strain, season to taste with salt, and pour the broth into jars. Cover and refrigerate for up to 5 days or freeze up to 3 months.

✚
Immune

Classic Mushroom-Vegetable Broth

While my seasonal broths are less for adding to recipes and more for sipping to keep me hydrated and healthy, this is my culinary broth of choice year-round. This savory mushroom broth is my go-to for most dishes. I add medicinal mushrooms like turkey tail and reishi for an immune system boost. You can use this recipe as an ingredient for any other recipe in this book that requires a mushroom broth.

MAKES: servings vary | PREP AND COOK TIME: 10 minutes, plus 4 to 24 hours to cook

1 pound mixed mushrooms, including shiitake, maitake, and cremini, roughly chopped

1-inch cube or 2 slices dried reishi mushrooms

2 or 3 dried turkey tail mushrooms

2 sprigs fresh rosemary

2 tablespoons fresh sage leaves, chopped

3 sprigs fresh thyme

4 sprigs fresh flat-leaf parsley

6 cloves garlic, smashed

1 large yellow onion, peeled and quartered

1 large carrot, peeled and roughly chopped

2 stalks celery with leaves, roughly chopped

10 black peppercorns

3 bay leaves

1. Place all the ingredients in slow cooker or large stock pot. Cover with water and bring to a simmer. Simmer for at least four hours on low heat, but preferably overnight. Season to taste with salt and pepper.

2. Let cool, strain, and pour into quart-size canning jars, leaving ½ inch of headspace at the top of each. Refrigerate for up to 5 days or freeze for up to 3 months.

✚ Adaptogenic, Immune

Roasted Ginger-Garlic Mushroom Broth

Roasting the mushrooms and other aromatics intensifies the flavor of this simple broth. Use it for Korean- or Japanese-inspired dishes, or simmer with additional medicinal mushrooms for a savory drink any time of day. Ginger shares potent anti-inflammatory and antioxidant properties, while garlic has both antimicrobial and antioxidant activity.

MAKES: servings vary | PREP AND COOK TIME: 10 minutes, plus 4 to 24 hours to cook

1 pound mixed fresh mushrooms (cremini, maitake, beech, white button, etc.), roughly chopped

2-inch piece fresh ginger, chopped

1 head garlic, broken into cloves but not peeled

1 onion, peeled and halved

1 ounce dried mushrooms, tough or tender

3 quarts water

1. Preheat the oven to 400°F. Line a baking sheet with parchment paper.

2. Place the fresh mushrooms, ginger, garlic, and onion on the prepared baking sheet. Roast for about 40 minutes, until nicely browned.

3. Transfer to a slow cooker or stock pot, along with any juices. Add the dried mushrooms and water.

4. Cook on high in a slow cooker for 8 hours, or bring to a simmer, then reduce heat to low and cook for 4 hours on the stovetop.

5. Let cool, strain, and pour into quart-size canning jars, leaving ½ inch of headspace at the top of each. Refrigerate for up to 5 days or freeze for up to 3 months.

✚ Immune

Shiitake-Kombu Miso Broth

Kombu is a seaweed—I prefer the term "sea vegetable"—so it's naturally cooling and moistening, with good mineral content. Once soaked and reconstituted, it becomes mucilaginous and will break down when cooked for hours, serving as a subtle, silky thickening agent. Kombu, which is said to strengthen the nervous system, has a very strong flavor that holds up well with shiitakes.

MAKES: servings vary | PREP AND COOK TIME: 10 minutes, plus 4 to 24 hours to cook

1 pound dried shiitake mushrooms, broken into pieces or roughly chopped

1 sheet kombu

1 leek or yellow onion, coarsely chopped

white miso paste, for serving

1. Place the mushrooms, kombu, and leek or onion in a slow cooker. Cover with water to the max-fill line. Cook on low for 8 hours or overnight. Strain. Cover and refrigerate for up to 5 days or freeze for up to 3 months.

2. Before serving, whisk 1 teaspoon white miso into each cup.

✚ Cholesterol, Detox, Immune, Nervous System, Skin

CHAPTER 11

Drinks and Elixirs

This is a chapter that leans more heavily on the tough than the tender mushrooms, in the form of extracts. These concentrated powders allow you to add mushrooms to any beverage, hot or cold. From lattes and teas—both with and without caffeine—to sports drinks, these recipes make integrating mushrooms in your daily routine delicious and easy. Some recipes simply add mushrooms to drinks you know and love, while others use mushroom extracts in unique new ways.

Slow Cooker Mushroom Tea

This is a basic recipe for mushroom tea, which is basically a mushroom extract; I like to use the slow cooker to make it easier. You can use a single mushroom or a combination. Evaporate more of the water by simmering it longer to create a stronger tea.

MAKES: servings vary | PREP AND COOK TIME: 10 minutes, plus 4 to 24 hours to cook

1 teaspoon chaga mushroom chunks or powdered mushroom (not powdered extract)

1 slice reishi mushroom or 1 teaspoon coarse reishi powder

1 turkey tail mushroom, crumbled, or 1 teaspoon coarse powder

Place your mushrooms in a slow cooker. Add water to the max-fill line (up to 2 liters). Cook on high overnight or up to 24 hours. Strain and drink as desired. Refrigerate for up to 5 days.

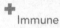

Immune

Turmeric-Ginger Chaga Tea

Hello, antioxidants! Free radicals don't stand a chance in the presence of turmeric, ginger, and chaga all in one mug. This is a tea that feels more healing that culinary in nature, but the taste is not unpleasant. I sip on it throughout winter (usually without sweetener).

SERVES: 1 | PREP TIME: 10 minutes

- 1 cup prepared chaga tea
- 1 teaspoon grated fresh turmeric
- 1 teaspoon grated fresh ginger
- 1 tablespoon honey or coconut sugar

Combine all the ingredients in a small saucepan over medium-low heat, and heat until simmering. Transfer to a mug and drink immediately.

+
Antioxidant, Immune

Tulsi-Ginger Reishi Tea

Tulsi, also known as holy basil in ayurveda, is sweet and fragrant. That it also helps me adapt to stress is a bonus. I drink at least one mug of tulsi tea daily, usually one of the Organic India blends. Tulsi and ginger is one of my favorite combinations, and I like adding reishi for a little extra calm.

SERVES: 1 | PREP TIME: 10 minutes

- 1 tulsi tea bag
- 1 tablespoon thinly sliced fresh ginger
- 1 teaspoon powdered reishi extract

Combine all the ingredients in a small saucepan over medium-low heat with 1 cup water. Simmer for at least 10 minutes. Strain out the ginger and serve immediately.

✚ Adaptogenic, Immune, Sleep, Stress

Can't Beet This Energy Drink

When it comes to energy, cordyceps and beets are a pair that, well, can't be beat. Put down the neon-colored cans of chemicals when you need a boost and instead reach for this natural, caffeine-free drink that's sweet, spicy, and tangy—and won't give you jitters. Include the apple for added sweetness.

SERVES: 1 | PREP TIME: 10 minutes

2 medium beets

3 medium carrots

1 medium apple (optional)

1 inch fresh turmeric

1 inch fresh ginger

1 serving powdered cordyceps extract

pinch of salt

Juice the beets, carrots, apple, if using, turmeric, and ginger. Stir in the cordyceps extract and a pinch of salt. Serve immediately, over ice if desired.

✚ Energy, Immune, Stress

Cordyceps–Coconut Water Sports Drink

As a hiker and runner who lives in the South, I need to supplement my workouts with electrolytes during summer months. In place of overly sweet sports drinks, I often use this coconut water–based drink. Coconut water contains some electrolytes, and I add a serving of electrolyte drops when I'll be out for more than 90 minutes (I like to use Elete Electrolytes). Orange and lime juice add vitamin C and flavor, and cordyceps supports energy while lion's mane helps with focus.

SERVES: 1 | PREP TIME: 10 minutes

12 ounces (1 ½ cups) coconut water

¼ cup fresh orange juice

1 tablespoon lime juice

pinch of sea salt or 1 serving electrolyte drops (optional)

1 teaspoon powdered cordyceps extract

1 teaspoon powdered lion's mane extract

Combine all ingredients in a blender, then transfer to a bottle.

✚ Energy, Immune

Ginger-Turmeric Elixir

Sip on this first thing in the morning to wake up your body and give your immune system some TLC. Lemon is cooling and astringent, which I find to be ideal for clearing morning congestion and stimulating digestion by causing you to salivate. Ginger and turmeric are always welcome in any elixir I make, and here they offer their one-two punch of antioxidant and anti-inflammatory support. I change up my immune mushroom blend based on what I have on hand.

SERVES: 1 | PREP TIME: 10 minutes

1 cup water

1 serving powdered mushroom extract (any combination of turkey tail, reishi, maitake, shiitake, cordyceps, and chaga)

½ teaspoon fresh grated ginger

1 teaspoon fresh grated turmeric

pinch of black pepper

juice of 1 lemon

honey or agave, to taste

1. Bring the water to a boil.

2. Place the mushroom powder in a large mug, then add a small amount of the boiling water and whisk to combine. Add the ginger, turmeric, pepper, and lemon juice, then pour in the rest of the water.

3. Let cool to desired temperature and drink immediately, adding honey or agave if desired.

✚
Adaptogenic, Digestion, Immune

Wellness Toddy

Sip on this spicy, tangy drink at the first sign of a tickle in your throat, or regularly throughout cold and flu season. Echinacea is a powerful immune-boosting herb, and you'll know yours is working when you feel its trademark tingle in your mouth. Skip the cayenne if you're sensitive to heat, but it really does help clear my sinuses. I pass on any added sweetener, but you can sweeten this drink to taste.

SERVES: 1 | PREP TIME: 10 minutes

1 cup water

1 serving powdered mushroom extract (any combination of turkey tail, reishi, maitake, shiitake, cordyceps, or chaga)

1 teaspoon fresh grated ginger

pinch of cayenne pepper (optional)

1 dropper echinacea tincture

juice of 1 lemon

honey or agave, to taste

1. Bring the water to a boil.

2. Place the mushroom powder in a large mug, then add a small amount of the boiling water and whisk to combine. Add the ginger, cayenne pepper, if using, echinacea, and lemon, then pour in the rest of the water.

3. Let cool to desired temperature and drink immediately, adding honey or agave if desired.

✚
Immune

Maple-Pecan Chaga Tea Latte

Maple and pecan are a lovely pairing. Pecans are a warming food that is said to support the nervous system, and I think they are highly underrated. Their subtle sweetness complements maple—my natural sweetener of choice—quite well. And I love the sweet nuttiness of maple-pecan milk with chaga tea. It just feels like a natural combination, since pecans, chaga, and maple all come from the woods!

SERVES: 1 | PREP AND COOK TIME: 5 minutes, plus overnight for the maple-pecan milk

For the maple-pecan milk:

½ cup pecans, soaked in water overnight

¾ cup water

1 vanilla bean or ¼ teaspoon vanilla powder

1 to 2 tablespoons maple syrup

pinch of sea salt

For the latte:

1 cup prepared chaga tea

1 tablespoon maple syrup

pinch of sea salt

1. To prepare the maple-pecan milk, drain and rinse the pecans, then add to a high-speed blender with 3/4 cup of water. Blend until smooth. Strain, reserving the pulp for another purpose, then return to the blender and add the vanilla, maple syrup, and salt. Process until frothy. Refrigerate for up to five days. Makes enough for four lattes.

2. To make the latte, heat the chaga tea with the maple and salt, then top with as much frothed milk as desired.

✚ Antioxidant, Immune

Mind-Boosting Matcha Latte

When I face a physically demanding day, I reach for coffee in the morning, despite my best efforts to limit it. But when my day appears it will be mentally taxing, I opt for matcha, usually with maca powder. This latte came about on a writing day when I wanted an extra boost of energy. Lion's mane provides concentration and focus, while cordyceps offers energy.

SERVES: 1 | PREP TIME: 10 minutes

2 teaspoons matcha powder

1 teaspoon maca powder

1 serving powdered cordyceps extract

1 serving powdered lion's mane extract

pinch of vanilla powder

1 teaspoon maple syrup or honey

8 ounces hot (but not boiling) water

1 teaspoon maple syrup or honey

up to ¼ cup frothed milk

1. Whisk together the matcha, maca, cordyceps and lion's mane extracts, and vanilla powder in a small bowl. (If you're using a traditional bamboo whisk, soak it in hot water first.)

2. Pour a small amount of hot water over the powders, and whisk until they form a paste. Add the maple syrup or honey. Continue to pour in the water in small amounts, whisking each time. Once all the water has been added, transfer to a mug, then top with the frothed milk.

✚ Adaptogenic, Energy, Immune, Memory, Nervous System

Turmeric Dirty Chai Mushroom Latte

This is a recipe for one of those mornings when you need energy, like, right now and throughout the day. Dirty lattes—with espresso and chai—are tasty and effectively caffeinated. This one has turmeric for its innumerable benefits as well as its bitter flavor, plus cordyceps for a different kind of energy. A bit of sweetness balances the drink.

SERVES: 1 | PREP TIME: 10 minutes

1 cup prepared chaga tea

1 black chai tea bag

1 serving powdered cordyceps extract

½ teaspoon dried turmeric

1 teaspoon honey or coconut sugar

1 shot prepared espresso

¼ cup frothed milk

1. In a saucepan on the stove, simmer the chaga tea with the chai tea bag for at least 10 minutes. Remove the tea bag.

2. Add the cordyceps extract and turmeric to a large mug, then add the sugar or honey, and whisk in the espresso. Carefully pour in the chaga chai, then top with the frothed milk. Drink immediately.

✚ Adaptogenic, Antioxidant, Immune

Iced Cinnamon Maitake Latte

This latte combines the top mushroom for blood sugar with two herbs that also help support healthy blood sugar levels, fenugreek and cinnamon. Fenugreek is commonly used in place of maple syrup (including in the artificially maple-flavored corn syrup) as they have a similar scent, and it pairs well with cinnamon.

SERVES: 1 | PREP TIME: 10 minutes

1 serving powdered maitake extract

½ teaspoon ground cinnamon

pinch of ground fenugreek

1 cup unsweetened vanilla soy or almond milk

1 cup prepared iced coffee or black tea

½ cup ice

Combine all the ingredients in a blender until icy and frothy. Transfer to a glass and drink immediately.

✚ Blood Sugar, Immune

Mind-Meld Mushroom Latte

You've likely heard of butter coffee by now. This is a dairy-free, mushroom-infused version. MCT oil is coconut oil that has had the solid-at-room-temperature fatty acids removed, leaving behind only those that are liquid. These medium-chain fatty acids are praised by fans of the ketogenic diet, who tout the oil's ability to provide energy and be more easily digested. You can use regular coconut oil if you prefer. Lion's mane and cordyceps are my favorite energy-boosting mushroom combo, so I always include them in my "mind-meld" lattes, whether I use matcha or coffee.

SERVES: 1 | PREP TIME: 10 minutes

- 1 cup hot brewed coffee or matcha
- 1 serving powdered cordyceps extract
- 1 serving powdered lion's mane extract
- 1 tablespoon coconut or MCT oil

Combine all the ingredients in a high-speed blender until smooth and frothy. Pour into a mug and drink immediately.

✚ Adaptogenic, Immune, Memory, Nervous System

Vanilla-Hemp Cordyceps Matcha Latte

Hemp is underrated as a food source, in my opinion, so I look for any opportunity to sneak hemp hearts into a recipe. Creamy when blended and tender when whole, they're packed with protein, fiber, and omega-3s. I sometimes make homemade hemp milk, but I usually just put everything into the blender (hemp hearts included) and give it a whirl.

SERVES: 1 | PREP TIME: 10 minutes

2 teaspoons matcha powder

1 serving powdered cordyceps extract

3 tablespoons hemp hearts

¼ teaspoon vanilla powder or extract

1 teaspoon maple syrup or honey

1½ cups water

Combine all the ingredients in a high-speed blender until smooth and frothy. Transfer to a small saucepan over medium heat. Bring to a simmer while whisking constantly. Pour into a mug and enjoy immediately.

+ Adaptogenic, Energy, Immune

Lavender-Peppermint Reishi Latte

Lavender and peppermint are a fragrant and delicious combination that calm and center the mind. Here, I've added reishi for a relaxing warm drink that's caffeine-free. I like to sip on this latte in the late afternoon when it's too close to bedtime for black or green tea and I want something more substantial than herbal tea.

SERVES: 1 | PREP TIME: 10 minutes

1 teaspoon powdered reishi extract

¼ teaspoon culinary-grade lavender

1 peppermint tea bag

1 teaspoon maple syrup or honey

up to ¼ cup frothed milk

1. Place the reishi, lavender, and peppermint tea bag in a large mug. Add hot but not boiling water, cover, and allow to steep for 10 minutes.

2. Stir in the maple syrup or honey, top with the frothed milk, and serve immediately.

✚ Adaptogenic, Immune, Sleep, Stress

Reishi-Turmeric Latte

I love turmeric in sweet and spicy drinks like this one. While it is bitter, it's also complexly earthy and fragrant, which I like in combination with spicy-sweet ginger, plus reishi—which should be bitter if it's potent. I like a little fat in this drink to help extract the fat-soluble components in the medicinal ingredients, as well as for mouthfeel.

SERVES: 1 | PREP TIME: 10 minutes

1 teaspoon powdered reishi extract

1 teaspoon grated fresh turmeric

1 teaspoon grated fresh ginger

1 pitted Medjool date

1 teaspoon coconut oil

pinch of sea salt

pinch of black pepper

½ cup water

1 cup almond or coconut milk

Combine all the ingredients in a high-speed blender, blending until smooth. Transfer to a small saucepan over medium-low heat, and heat until simmering. Transfer to a mug and drink immediately.

Adaptogenic, Immune, Sleep, Stress

Memory Matcha Latte

Working from home means I can get creative with beverages throughout the day. This matcha latte takes a bit more work than a simple cup of tea, but it's worth every second (and still takes just 10 minutes). Peppermint is naturally stimulating, tulsi (holy basil) is fragrant and supports stress management, and both gotu kola and ginkgo biloba are classic brain-boosting herbs that promote healthy circulation. Add lion's mane, and you'll be ready for whatever task is next on your to-do list.

SERVES: 1 | PREP TIME: 10 minutes

1 peppermint tea bag

1 tulsi tea bag

1 teaspoon matcha powder

1 serving powdered lion's mane extract

1 teaspoon sweetener of choice

¼ cup milk

1 dropper gotu kola tincture (optional)

1 dropper ginkgo biloba tincture (optional)

1. Steep the tea bags in hot water for at least 10 minutes in a small saucepan or teapot.

2. Meanwhile, whisk together the matcha, lion's mane, sweetener, milk, and tinctures in a mug. Carefully pour the hot tea into the mug and serve immediately.

✚
Energy, Immune, Memory, Stress,

Reishi Vanilla-Cardamom Latte

A little cardamom goes a long way, and in this recipe, it is assertive yet not overpowering. The vanilla in this naturally-sweetened almond milk latte tames the bitterness of reishi. Serve this caffeine-free drink after a large, heavy evening meal.

SERVES: 1 | PREP TIME: 10 minutes

1 teaspoon powdered reishi extract

¼ teaspoon vanilla powder

¼ teaspoon ground cardamom

½ cup water

1 cup almond milk

1 teaspoon sweetener of choice

Combine the reishi, vanilla, cardamom, and water and the almond milk in a small saucepan over medium-low heat. Let simmer for 10 minutes, then stir in sweetener, and serve immediately.

✚ Adaptogenic, Immune, Sleep, Stress

Nutella Mushroom Mocha

Nutella mochas are heaven in a cup, and if you add mushrooms, they're even better, in my opinion. With coffee, plus lion's mane and cordyceps, this mocha is sure to perk you up. I firmly believe you can't have a bad day if you start your morning with one of these.

SERVES: 1 | PREP TIME: 10 minutes

1 serving powdered lion's mane extract

1 serving powdered cordyceps extract

1 tablespoon Nutella or another chocolate-hazelnut spread

1 cup prepared coffee

¼ cup almond milk

Combine all the ingredients in a blender, blending until completely smooth. If desired, heat in a small saucepan over medium-low heat until simmering. Drink immediately.

✚ Adaptogenic, Energy, Immune, Memory, Stress

Chaga Orange-Ginger Hot Chocolate

Orange and ginger are two of my favorite ingredients to pair with chocolate, and they're the predominant flavors in this chaga hot chocolate. I use a combo of coconut and almond milk for richness, plus a date for natural sweetness. This is not quite as rich as sipping chocolate, though it comes close. Keep stirring the hot chocolate as you sip it, to ensure the good stuff doesn't get left in the bottom of your mug.

SERVES: 1 | PREP TIME: 10 minutes

1 cup almond milk

½ cup coconut milk

1 pitted Medjool date

1 serving powdered chaga extract

2 tablespoons chopped bittersweet chocolate

2 tablespoons dark cocoa powder

¼ teaspoon vanilla extract

1 teaspoon orange zest

2 tablespoons orange juice

1 teaspoon grated fresh ginger

pinch of sea salt

Combine all the ingredients in a high-speed blender, blending until smooth. Transfer to a small saucepan over medium-low heat, and heat until simmering. Transfer to a mug and drink immediately.

✚ Antioxidant, Immune

Reishi Peppermint Hot Chocolate

The bitterness of reishi plus the cooling tingle of peppermint make this hot chocolate a winner. It's naturally sweetened with a date, but you can swap in stevia or another sweetener if desired. You can change up the milks, but use one that has some heft to it. You want a little fat for satiety in this drink.

SERVES: 1 | PREP tIME: 10 minutes to prepare and cook

1 cup almond milk

½ cup coconut milk

1 teaspoon powdered reishi extract

2 tablespoons chopped bittersweet chocolate

2 tablespoons dark cocoa powder

1 pitted date

2 droppers peppermint tincture or ¼ teaspoon peppermint extract

pinch of sea salt

Combine all the ingredients in a high-speed blender, blending until smooth. Transfer to a small saucepan over medium-low heat, and heat until simmering. Transfer to a mug and drink immediately.

✚ Adaptogenic, Immune, Mood, Sleep, Stress

Chaga Chai

Chaga chai is a classic preparation for this immune-boosting mushroom. This version is simple, using a premeasured blend. I buy a mix from my favorite tea shop, Dobra, but you can swap in a decaffeinated chai tea bag if desired.

SERVES: 1 | PREP TIME: 10 minutes

1 cup chaga tea

1 teaspoon chai spices

maple syrup or honey, to taste

2 tablespoons coconut milk

1. In a small saucepan over medium-low heat, simmer the chaga tea with the chai spices for at least 10 minutes.

2. Strain the tea into a mug, then add the maple syrup or honey to taste and whisk in the coconut milk. Serve immediately.

+
Antioxidant, Immune

Golden Milk with Chaga

Creamy, turmeric-based golden milk is a delightfully nourishing beverage. During my time working in the supplements industry, I spent a lot of time serving up this sunny yellow drink. I have a soft spot for it, but I now tire easily of the classic, so I often change it up. I keep my base recipe simple: turmeric, vanilla, black pepper (to aid absorption of turmeric), plus coconut milk and a tiny bit of sweetener. This time I added chaga to infuse this cozy beverage with some mushroom goodness.

SERVES: 1 | PREP TIME: 10 minutes

1 cup chaga tea

2 teaspoons grated fresh turmeric

1 tablespoon honey or coconut sugar

1 teaspoon coconut oil

pinch of vanilla powder

pinch of sea salt

pinch of pepper

¼ cup coconut milk

Combine all the ingredients in a high-speed blender, blending until smooth. Transfer to a small saucepan over medium-low heat, and heat until simmering. Transfer to a mug and drink immediately.

✚ Antioxidant, Immune

Warm Reishi Milk

This is the grown-up version of the warm milk we sipped before bedtime as kids. It tastes like a hug in a mug. The reishi is bitter but blends into the creamy milk, and a bit of sweetness helps to balance the flavor. Nutmeg is the fragrant, comforting, proverbial cherry on top. I love curling up in bed with this milk and my journal as a gentle way to wind down a long day.

SERVES: 1 | PREP TIME: 10 minutes

1 cup reishi tea or 1 cup water with 1 serving powdered reishi extract

¼ cup milk

1 teaspoon maple syrup, or to taste

⅛ teaspoon ground nutmeg

In a small saucepan over medium-low heat, bring all the ingredients to a simmer, then let steep for 10 minutes. Drink immediately.

✚ Adaptogenic, Immune, Sleep, Stress

Shiitake Bloody Mary

Sometimes you have to have a little fun with mushrooms. Once I made Shiitake Vodka ("Chanterelle or Shiitake Vodka" on page 197), I needed to use it, so I made this Bloody Mary—with extra shiitake powder, of course. Everyone has a secret ingredient to make this classic tomato juice cocktail stand out. Mine is kimchi juice—the liquid in the bottom of the kimchi jar (or any fermented vegetables I have in the fridge). It adds tanginess and probiotics. I use Mushroom Soy Sauce, but you can swap in plain soy sauce or aminos if you only have that.

SERVES: 1 | PREP TIME: 10 minutes

½ cup tomato juice

1½ ounces vodka or Shiitake Vodka ("Chanterelle or Shiitake Vodka" on page 197)

1 serving shiitake or powdered maitake extract

juice of 1 lemon

1 tablespoon kimchi or sauerkraut juice

½ teaspoon Mushroom Soy Sauce ("Mushroom Soy Sauce" on page 202)

¼ teaspoon ground celery seed

hot sauce, to taste

salt and pepper, to taste

Fill a shaker with ice and add all the ingredients. Shake to combine. Serve immediately, garnished as desired, with fresh or pickled vegetables.

✚ Beauty, Cholesterol, Detox, Immune

Notes

1. Christopher Hobbs, *Medicinal Mushrooms: An Exploration of Healing, Tradition, and Culture*, Summertown, TN: Book Pub, 2003.

2. Broderick Parr, et al., "Flooding, Hurricanes, and Drought Disrupt Otherwise Strong Vegetable and Dry Pulse Markets," *Vegetables and Pulses Outlook* (October 2017), https://www.ers.usda.gov/webdocs/publications/85540/vgs-359.pdf?v=43035.

3. William K. Stevens, "Rearranging the Branches on a New Tree of Life," *New York Times*, August 31, 1999, https://www.nytimes.com/1999/08/31/science/rearranging-the-branches-on-a-new-tree-of-life.html.

4. American Psychological Association, "APA *Stress in America Survey*: US at 'Lowest Point We Can Remember;' Future of Nation Most Commonly Reported Source of Stress," November 1, 2017, http://www.apa.org/news/press/releases/2017/11/lowest-point.aspx.

5. American Psychological Association, "Stress About Health Insurance Costs Reported by Majority of Americans, APA *Stress in America* Survey Reveals," January 24, 2018, http://www.apa.org/news/press/releases/2018/01/insurance-costs.aspx

6. Ronald Glaser and Janice Kiecolt-Glaser, "Stress-Induced Immune Disfunction: Implications for Health," *Nature Reviews Immunology* 5, no. 3 (March 2005): 243–51, doi: 10.1038/nri1571.

7. Anxiety and Depression Association of America, "Facts and Statistics," https://adaa.org/about-adaa/press-room/facts-statistics#.

8. Aaron Lerner, Patricia Jeremias, et al., "The World Incidence and Prevalence of Autoimmune Diseases is Increasing," *International Journal of Celiac Disease* 3, no. 4: 151–55, doi: 10.12691/ijcd-3-4-8.

9. Flavio A. Cadegiani and Claudio E. Kater, "Adrenal Fatigue Does Not Exist: A Systematic Review," *BMC Endocrine Disorders* 16, no. 1 (2016), doi: 10.1186/s12902-016-0128-4.

10. Hobbs.

11. Hobbs.

12. Michael d'Estries, "11 Things You May Not Know About Otzi the Iceman," *Mother Nature Network*, August 21, 2016. Retrieved from https://www.mnn.com/lifestyle/arts-culture/blogs/11-things-you-dont-know-about-otzi.

13. The Mushroom Council, "FAQ," https://www.mushroomcouncil.com/faq.

14. SPINS, "Top 10 Trend Predictions for 2018," http://www.spins.com/wp-content/uploads/2018/01/TrendWatch-2018TrendPredictions.pdf.

15. Cheryl Dikeman, Laura Bauer, et al., "Effects of Stage of Maturity and Cooking on the Chemical Composition of Select Mushroom Varieties," *Journal of Agricultural and Food Chemistry 53*, no. 4 (January 2005): 1130-1138, doi: 10.1021/jf048541l.

16. Peter Roupas, Jennifer Keough, et al, "Mushrooms and Agaritine: A Mini-Review," *Journal of Functional Foods* 2, no. 2 (April 2010): 91–98, doi: 10.1016/j.jff.2010.04.003.

17. Hobbs.

18. Michael W. Beug, "Shiitake Dermatitis Alert," *North American Mycological Association*, https://www.namyco.org/shiitake_dermatitis.php.

19. Lawrence Cheskin, Lisa Davis, et al., "Lack of Energy Compensation Over 4 Days When White Button Mushrooms Are Substituted for Beef," *Appetite* 51 (2008): 50–57, doi: 10.1016/j.appet.2007.11.007.

20. Ralph H. Kurtzman, "Nutrition from Mushrooms, Understanding and Reconciling Available Data," *Mycoscience* 38, no. 2 (July 1997): 247–53, doi: 10.1007/BF02460860.

21. Hobbs.

22. Hobbs.

23. The Mushroom Council, "Vitamin D," https://www.mushroomcouncil.com/vitamin-d/.

24. USDA, "Dietary Guidelines for Americans, 2015–2020, Eighth Edition," https://health.gov/dietaryguidelines/2015/resources/2015-2020_Dietary_Guidelines.pdf.

25. Fumio Watanabe, Yukinori Yabuta, et al., "Vitamin B12-Containing Plant Food Sources for Vegetarians," *Nutrients* 6 no. 5 (May 2014): 1861–73, doi: 10.3390/nu6051861.

26. Roberta Larson Duyff, *Academy of Nutrition and Dietetics Complete Food and Nutrition Guide*, 5th Ed. New York: Academy of Nutrition and Dietetics, 2017.

27. N. Joy Dubost, et al., "Identification and Quantification of Ergothioneine in Cultivated Mushrooms by Liquid Chromatography-Mass Spectroscopy," *International Journal of Medicinal Mushrooms* 8 (2006): 215–22, doi: 10.1615/IntJMedMushr.v8.i3.30.

28. Michael Kalaras, John Richie, et al., "Mushrooms: A Rich Source of the Antioxidants Ergothioneine and Glutathione," *Food Chemistry* 233 (October 2017): 429–33, doi: 10.1615/IntJMedMushr.v8.i3.30.

29. Harry Marsales, B. T. Williams, et al., "The Effect of Mushroom Intake on Modulating Post-Prandial Glycemic Response," *The FASEB Journal* 28, no. 1 suppl. (April 2014).

30. Mona Calvo, et al., "Risk Factor Modification in Pre-Diabetic Adults Consuming White Button Mushrooms Rich in the Anti-Oxidant Ergothioneine," *The FASEB Journal* 28, no. 1 suppl. (April 2014).

31. A. Shin, et al., "Dietary Mushroom Intake and the Risk of Breast Cancer Based on Hormone Receptor Status," *Nutrition and Cancer* 62, no. 4 (2010): 476–83; S. Zang, Y. Tomata, K. Sugiyama, Y. Sugawara, and I. Tsuji, "Mushroom Consumption and Incident Dementia in Elderly Japanese: The Ohsaki Cohort 2006 Study," Journal of the American Geriatrics Society 65, no. 7 (July 2017): 1462–69.

32. R. Chang, "Functional Properties of Edible Mushrooms," *Nutrition Review* 54, no. 11 part 2 (November 1996): S91–93.

33. U.S. Department of Agriculture, Agricultural Research Service, USDA Nutrient Data Laboratory, 2009; USDA National Nutrient Database for Standard Reference, www.ars.usda.gov/nutrientdata; N. J. Dubost et al., "Identification and Quantification of Ergothioneine in Cultivated Mushrooms by Liquid Chromatography-Mass Spectroscopy," *International Journal of Medicinal Mushrooms* 8 (2006): 215–22; The Mushroom Council, "Versatility in Varieties," Retrieved from https://www.mushroomcouncil.com/wp-content/uploads/2017/12/Versatility-in-Varieties.pdf

34. Hobbs.

35. Feng Hong, Jun Yan, et al., "Mechanism by Which Orally Administered Beta-1,3-Glucans Enhance the Tumoricidal Activity of Antitumor Monoclonal Antibodies in Murine Tumor Models," *Journal of Immunology* 173, no. 2 (July 2004): 797–806, doi: https://doi.org/10.4049/jimmunol.173.2.797. Z. Konopski, J. Fandrem, R. Seljelid, and T. Eskeland, "Interferon-Gamma Inhibits Endocytosis of Soluble Aminated ß-l,3-D-Glucan and Neutral Red in Mouse Peritoneal Macrophages," *Journal of Interferon and Cytokine Research* 15, no. 7 (July 1995): 597–603.

36. Hobbs.

37. Alexander Panossian and Georg Wikman, "Effects of Adaptogens on the Central Nervous System and the Molecular Mechanisms Associated with Their Stress-Protective Activity," *Pharmaceuticals* 3, no. 1 (January 2010): 188–224, doi: 10.3390/ph3010188.

38. David Winston and Steven Maimes, *Adaptogens: Herbs for strength, stamina, and stress relief.* (Rochester, VT: Healing Arts Press, 2007).

39. April Fulton, "Mushrooms Are Good for You, but Are They Medicine?" *Morning Edition*, National Public Radio, February 5, 2018, https://www.npr.org/sections/thesalt/2018/02/05/581917882/mushrooms-are-good-for-you-but-are-they-medicine.

40. Hobbs.

41. Robert Rogers, *The Fungal Pharmacy: The Complete Guide to Medicinal Mushrooms and Lichens of North America,* (Berkeley, CA: North Atlantic Books, 2011.)

42. Rogers.

43. Rogers.

44. Hobbs.

45. Hobbs.

46. Rogers.

47. Rogers.

48. Nuhu Alam, Ki Nam Yoon, et al., "Dietary Effect of Pleurotus Eryngii on Biochemical Function and Histology In Hypercholesterolemic Rats," *Saudi Journal of Biological Sciences* 18, no. 4 (October 2011): 403–409, doi: 10.1016/j.sjbs.2011.07.001.

49. Dan Charles, "How a Sleepy Pennsylvania Town Grew Into America's Mushroom Capital," National Public Radio, October 11, 2012, https://www.npr.org/sections/thesalt/2012/10/12/162719130/how-a-sleepy-pennsylvania-town-grew-into-americas-mushroom-capital.

50. Rogers.

51. "Dirty Dozen: EWG's 2018 Shopper's Guide to Pesticides in Produce," EWG, https://www.ewg.org/foodnews/dirty-dozen.php.

52. Gillian Harris and Helen Coulthard, "Early Eating Behaviours and Food Acceptance Revisited: Breastfeeding and Introduction of Complementary Foods as Predictive of Food Acceptance," *Current Obesity Reports* 5 (2016): 113–20, doi: 10.1007/s13679-016-0202-2.

53. Andrea Maier, Claire Chabanet, et al., "Effects of Repeated Exposure on Acceptance of Initially Disliked Vegetables in 7-Month Old Infants," Food Quality and Preference 18, no 8 (December 2007): 1023–32.

54. Hobbs.

55. Bee Wilson, "Yes, Bacon Really Is Killing Us," *The Guardian*, March 1, 2018, https://www.theguardian.com/news/2018/mar/01/bacon-cancer-processed-meats-nitrates-nitrites-sausages.

56. World Health Organization, "Q&A on the Carcinogenicity of the Consumption of Red Meat and Processed Meat," October 2015, Retrieved from http://www.who.int/features/qa/cancer-red-meat/en/.

57. Rogers.

58. Sandra Amalie Lacoppidan, et al., "Adherence to a Healthy Nordic Food Index Is Associated with a Lower Risk of Type-2 Diabetes—The Danish Diet, Cancer and Health Cohort Study," *Nutrients* 7, no. 10 (October 2015) 8633–64, doi: 10.3390/nu7105418.

59. A. Mydral Miller et al., "Flavor-Enhancing Properties of Mushrooms in Meat-Based Dishes in Which Sodium Has Been Reduced and Meat Has Been Partially Substituted with Mushrooms," *Journal of Food Science* 79, no. 9 (August 2014): S1795–S1804, doi: 10.1111/1750-3841.

60. E. A. Al-Dujaili, C. J. Kenyon, M. R. Nicol, and J. I. Mason., "Liquorice and Glycyrrhetinic Acid Increase DHEA and Deoxycorticosterone Levels In Vivo and In Vitro by Inhibiting Adrenal SULT2A1 Activity," *Molecular and Cellular Endocrinology* 336, no. 1-2 (April 2011): 102–109, doi: 10.1016 /j.mce.2010.12.011.

61. Astrid Nehlig, "The Neuroprotective Effects of Cocoa Flavanol and Its Influence on Cognitive Performance," *British Journal of Clinical Pharmacology* 75, no. 3 (March 2013): 716–27, doi: 10.1111/j.1365-2125.2012.04378.x.

62. Michael Gregor, "Is Mornia (*Moringa oleifera*) Good for You?" NutritionFacts .org, November 8, 2012, https://nutritionfacts.org/questions/ the-health-benefits-of-moringa/.

63. Giana Angelo, "Essential Fatty Acids and Skin Health," Linus Pauling Institute, Oregon State University, February 2012, http://lpi.oregonstate.edu/ mic/health-disease/skin-health/essential-fatty-acids.

64. University of Exeter, "Blueberry Concentrate Improves Brain Function in Older Adults," *ScienceDaily*, March 7, 2017, https://www.sciencedaily.com/ releases/2017/03/170307100356.htm.

65. Valentina Socci, Daniela Tempesta, et al., "Enhancing Human Cognition with Cocoa Flavonoids," *Frontiers in Nutrition* 4, no. 19 (May 2017), doi: 10.3389/ fnut.2017.00019

66. Tony Amidor, "Ask the Expert: Tart Cherry Juice and Exercise Recovery," *Today's Dietitian* 17, no. 11 (November 2015): 8, http://www.todaysdietitian .com/newarchives/1115p8.shtml.

67. Monica Reinagel, "Carob vs. Chocolate," *QuickandDirtyTips.com*, October 22, 2013, https://www.quickanddirtytips.com/health-fitness/healthy-eating/ carob-vs-chocolate.

68. Kerstin Iffland and Franjo Grotenhemen, "An Update on Safety and Side Effects of Cannabidiol: A Review of Clinical Data and Relevant Animal Studies," *Cannabis and Cannabinoid Research* 2, no. 1 (2017): 139–57, doi: 10.1089/ can.2016.0034.

69. "In the journals: Cocoa reduces inflammation assocaited with heart disease," *Harvard Woman's Health Watch*, February 2010, https://www.health.harvard .edu/newsletter_article/cocoa-reduces-inflammation-associated-with-heart -disease.

Selected Sources

Bone, Eugenia. *Mycophilia: Revelations from the Weird World of Mushrooms*. New York: Rodale, 2011.

Child, Julia, Louise Bertholle, and Simone Beck. *Mastering the Art of French Cooking*. New York: Alfred A. Knopf, 2016.

Czarnecki, Jack. *A Cook's Book of Mushrooms: With 100 Recipes for Common and Uncommon Varieties*. New York: Artisan, 1995.

Farges, Amy. *The Mushroom Lover's Mushroom Cookbook and Primer*. New York: Workman, 2000.

Gladstar, Rosemary. *Herbs for Long-Lasting Health: How to Make and Use Herbal Remedies for Lifelong Vitality*. North Adams, MA: Storey, 2014.

Greger, Michael. *How Not to Die: Discover the Foods Scientifically Proven to Prevent and Reverse Disease*. New York: Flatiron, 2015.

Herbst, Ron, and Sharon Tyler Herbst. *The New Food Lover's Companion*. Hauppauge, NY: Barrons Educational Series, 2007.

Hobbs, Christopher. *Medicinal Mushrooms: An Exploration of Healing, Tradition, and Culture*. Summertown, TN: Book Pub, 2003.

Isokauppila, Tero. *Healing Mushrooms: A Practical and Culinary Guide to Using Mushrooms for Whole Body Health*. New York: Avery, 2017.

Pitchford, Paul. *Healing with Whole Foods: Asian Traditions and Modern Nutrition*. Berkeley, CA: North Atlantic Books, 2009.

Rogers, Robert. *The Fungal Pharmacy: The Complete Guide to Medicinal Mushrooms and Lichens of North America*. Berkeley, CA: North Atlantic Books, 2011.

Selengut, Becky. *Shroom: Mind-Bendingly Good Recipes for Cultivated and Wild Mushrooms*. Kansas City, MO: Andrews McMeel, 2014.

Stamets, Paul. *Growing Gourmet and Medicinal Mushrooms: A Companion Guide to the Mushroom Cultivator*. Berkeley, CA: Ten Speed, 1994

Stamets, Paul. Mycelium Running: *How Mushrooms Can Help Save the World*. Berkeley, CA: Ten Speed, 2005.

Wang, Yuan, Warren Sheir, and Mika Ono. *Ancient Wisdom, Modern Kitchen: Recipes from the East for Health, Healing, and Long Life*. Cambridge, MA: Da Capo Lifelong, 2010

Winston, David, and Steven Maimes. *Adaptogens: Herbs for Strength, Stamina, and Stress Relief*. Rochester, VT: Healing Arts, 2007.

Wood, Rebecca. *The Whole Foods Encyclopedia: A Shopper's Guide*. New York: Prentice Hall, 1988.

Resources

For learning more about mushrooms, foraging, and a plant-based lifestyle, the author recommends the following sites:

Pisgah Gourmet, a grower of culinary and medicinal mushrooms: https://pisgahgourmet.com

No Taste Like Home, foraging and harvesting tours: https://notastelikehome.org

Becky Beyer, foraging and Appalachian lifestyle: http://www.bloodandspicebush.com

Abby Artemisia's WANDER (Wild Artemisia Nature Discovery, Empowerment, and Reconnection) School, http://www.thewanderschool.com

The following brands offer recommended mushroom- and plant-based products. Many recipes in this book were made using products from these brands.

- Emerald Cove
- Emperor's Kitchen
- Hodo Soy
- Manitoba Harvest
- Miso Master
- Om Organic Mushroom Powders
- Smiling Hara Hempeh
- Real Mushrooms

Recipe Index

Acknowledgments

The author would like to thank:

Sam, for always being the best.

My YAM fam, for giving me a soft place to land when I needed it most, and my YAM students, for enthusiastically testing every bite, ball, and treat in this book!

Jenna and Beth, for your unrivaled enthusiasm and kindness.

Ali and the team at Bounty and Soul: A portion of the proceeds from this book will go to Bounty and Soul, a grassroots, volunteer-run nonprofit that provides healthy food, nutrition education, and other resources to underserved communities in Buncombe County, North Carolina, ensuring that health and healthy eating are not a luxury, but a right. All donations will go toward providing plant-based and, of course, mushroom-based foods!

Dr. Mary Bove, for your encouragement and wisdom, especially for this book.

My recipe testers, including my mom, Jessica Grosman, and my dear friend Laura Arenschield.

Abby Artemisia, for your support and for the recipes you contributed.

The experts who've inspired my love of mushrooms, both those who spoke to me for this book and those who've shared their wisdom at conferences, on foraging trips, and via their blogs and Instagram feeds, including Eric Christianson of Pisgah Gourmet, the members of Food Fight Farm, Alan Muskat, Becky Beyer, Nate Burrows, and Skye Chilton.

About the Author

Stepfanie Romine has lived and cooked on three continents. A trained journalist, Stepfanie has worked as editorial director for an online healthy living community, and as a copywriter and recipe developer for an herbal products manufacturer. She is an editor and writer specializing in plant-based nutrition and natural health and wellness, and she also teaches yoga and cooking classes.

Stepfanie was introduced to mushrooms during her travels. Then in 2012, she and her husband Sam moved to the mountains of North Carolina to prioritize healthy living. A temperate rainforest with unparalleled biodiversity, Asheville and the surrounding area is a mecca for natural health, and Stepfanie dove right in, learning about herbal medicine, foraging for plants and mushrooms, and soaking up as much information about the natural world as possible. Having followed a plant-based diet since 2010, Stepfanie felt drawn to natural and herbal medicine, including the healing power of mushrooms.

Stepfanie is an experienced registered yoga teacher, and she is also a certified health coach and fitness nutrition specialist. She also taken courses in herbal supplements and holistic and integrative nutrition.

Stepfanie cooks healthy, seasonal plant-based meals (with plenty of mushrooms) to fuel her active life and her husband's long-distance road cycling. Stepfanie is the co-author of three books, most recently *The No Meat Athlete Cookbook.* Find her online at www.theflexiblekitchen.com. She lives in the mountains of Western North Carolina.